THE COMPLET
KETO DIET CO

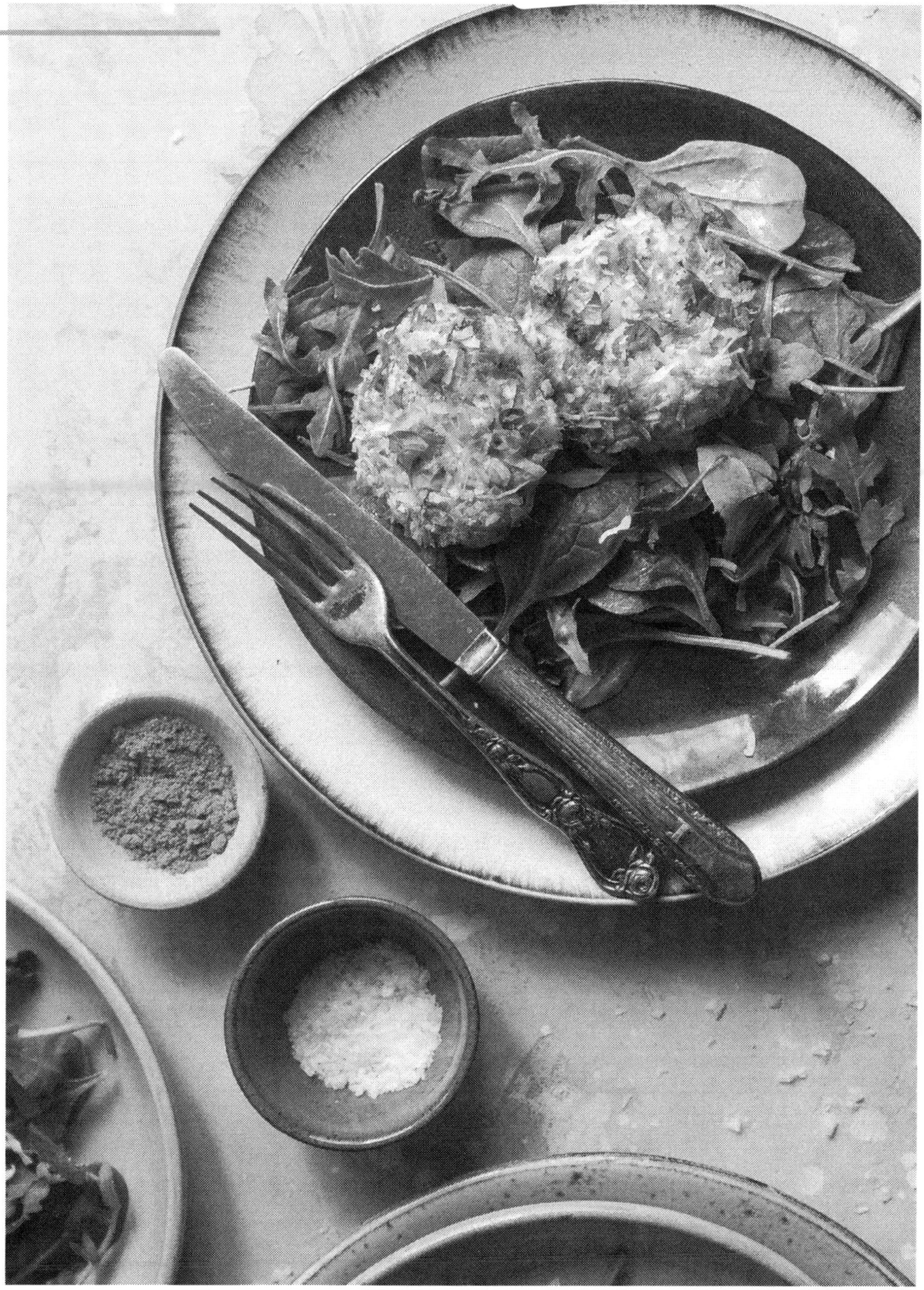

Jerry Carr

LEGAL & DISCLAIMER

The information contained in this book and its contents is not designed to replace or take the place of any form of medical or professional advice; and is not meant to replace the need for independent medical, financial, legal, or other professional advice or services, as may be required. The content and information in this book have been provided for educational and entertainment purposes only.

The content and information contained in this book have been compiled from sources deemed reliable, and it is accurate to the best of the Author's knowledge, information, and belief.

However, the author cannot guarantee its accuracy and validity and cannot be held liable for any errors and/or omissions. Further, changes are periodically made to this book as and when needed.

Where appropriate and/or necessary, you must consult a professional (including but not limited to your doctor, attorney, financial advisor, or such other professional advisor) before using any of the suggested remedies, techniques, or information in this book.

Upon using the contents and information contained in this book, you agree to hold harmless the Author from and against any damages, costs, and expenses, including any legal fees potentially resulting from the application of any of the information provided by this book. This disclaimer applies to any loss, damages, or injury caused by the use and application, whether directly or indirectly, of any advice or information presented, whether for breach of contract, tort, negligence, personal injury, criminal intent, or under any other cause of action. You agree to accept all risks of using the information presented inside this book.You agree that by continuing to read this book, where appropriate and/or necessary, you shall consult a professional (including but not limited to your doctor, attorney, or financial advisor, or such other advisor as needed) before using any of the suggested remedies, techniques, or information in this book.

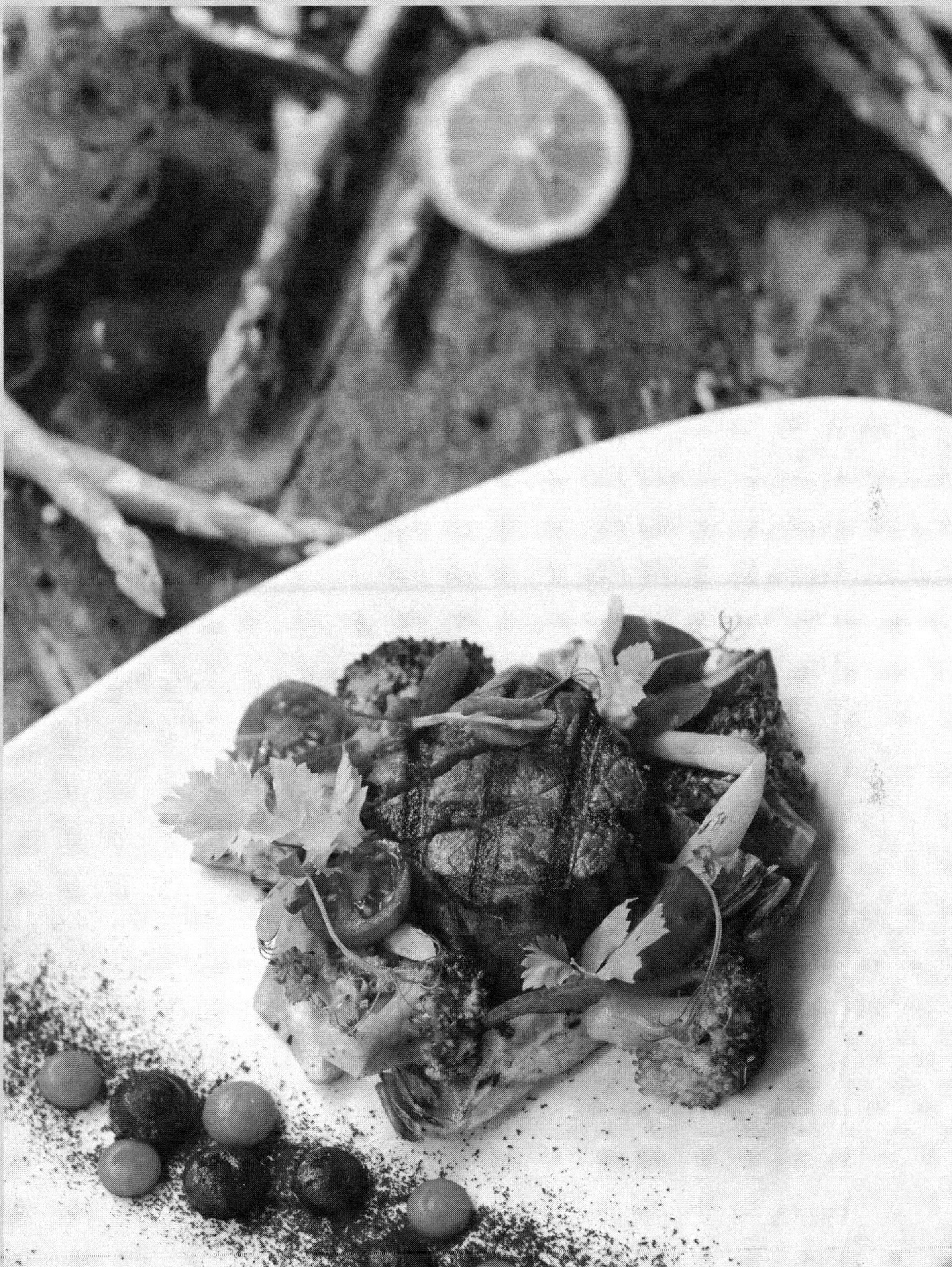

TABLE OF CONTENT

INTRODUCTION

This book is designed in a way that is easy to understand, about the secrets of the ketogenic diet, ketosis, and the countless health benefits associated with this lifestyle change. Ketogenic diets have been used for thousands of years for their many health benefits, ease of implementation, and simply because of the environments we evolved in.

Surprisingly, the Ketogenic diet was not created as a weight loss system. Instead, it was originally designed as an effective way to inhibit seizures in epileptic patients. It is intended to make sure the body gets enough protein and nutrients to stay healthy and energized, but not so many that it gains weight.

Over the years, as the diet gained in popularity, it began to be used for additional therapies, including the treatment of rare metabolic diseases, brain tumors, autism, depression, migraine headaches, and even Type 2 Diabetes. It has also been used for traumatic brain injuries, strokes, Parkinson's, and Alzheimer's disease. Oncologists even recommends this diet to cancer patients.

Because this diet works to improve health, while also decreasing weight, it has become a popular choice for everyone who wishes to lose weight, live a healthy lifestyle, or both. It is the best way to rapidly lose weight, without sacrificing your health or taking harmful drugs.

The Ketogenic diet is very scientific in how it works. It is designed to put the body in a state of ketosis. This state is reached when your body starts burning fat stores for fuel, instead of sugars. As you can imagine, burning the storage of fat is exactly what you need to do in order to lose the type of weight that you really want to lose, while maintaining your muscles.

Along with burning fat stores, ketosis has a neurological effect that will leave you feeling happier and less hungry. Both of these results will further help you lose any amount of weight you want. Because it is a healthy way to eat, you can continue with the Ketogenic diet indefinitely in order to maintain the ideal weight for your body type. At the completion of this book, you will have a much better understanding of the Keto diet and be able to experiment with the different recipes.

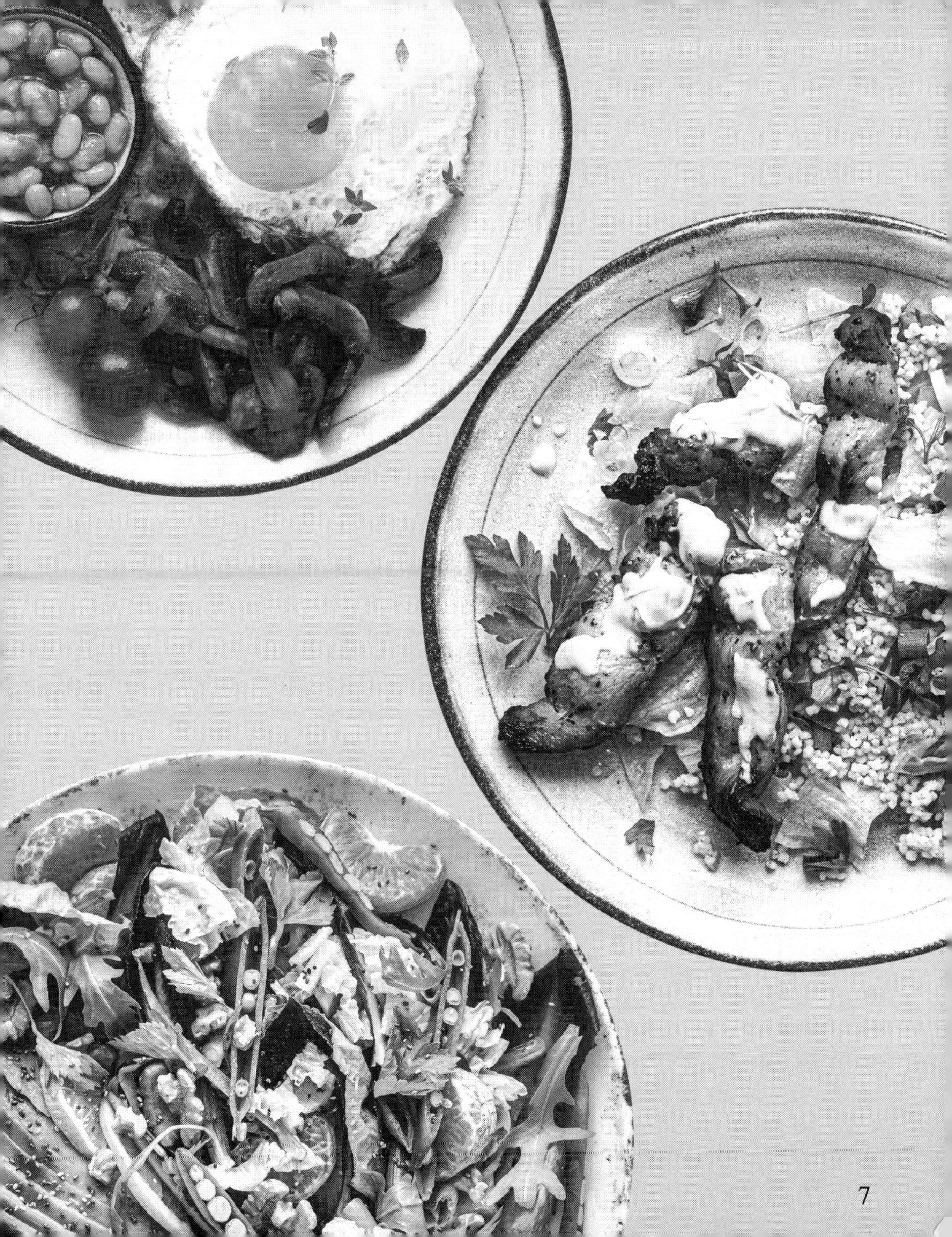

HOW DOES THE KETOGENIC DIET WORK?

We all know that we need energy food. On a typical high-carb diet, your body specifically uses glucose as the primary energy source; it is easier for your body to convert carbs to glucose than it is with other types of energy sources.

Insulin will also be produced to process the glucose in your bloodstream, and the fats will get stored by the body, eventually piling up and causing a litany of health problems.

The ketogenic diet enables your body to use another energy source for fuel; the concept is that with a lower carb intake, you will be depriving your body of the glucose it needs and will make use of the fats instead, as it falls into a state known as ketosis.

Ketosis is a natural state of the body wherein the liver will break down the available fats instead of glucose or carbohydrates, and ketones will be produced, which will then be burned by the body as the primary energy source; your goal with the ketogenic diet is to force your body into this metabolic state.

Your body is designed to adapt to a metabolic state easily, so you only need to worry about following the diet and let your body handle the rest.

The ketogenic diet is different from other low-carb diets. The difference is that your diet should be about 70-75 percent of calories from fat, 20-25 percent from protein, and 5-10 percent from carbohydrates each day.

If you follow these guidelines, your diet will be composed of high-fats and moderate protein intake, and there will be no need to count calories.

Protein is limited because it affects the insulin and blood sugar in your body.

If you consume protein in large quantities, the excess gets converted to glucose. As a result, your body will not reach a state of ketosis. Have you ever come to note that whenever you have a food craving, you usually go for carb-rich foods? That's because your brain has labeled starchy and sweet foods as comfort foods. Our main goal with the ketogenic diet is to drastically reduce the intake of carbohydrates and choose a healthier alternative.In theory, if you limit your carb intake and achieve a state of ketosis, the excess weight will be shed easily.

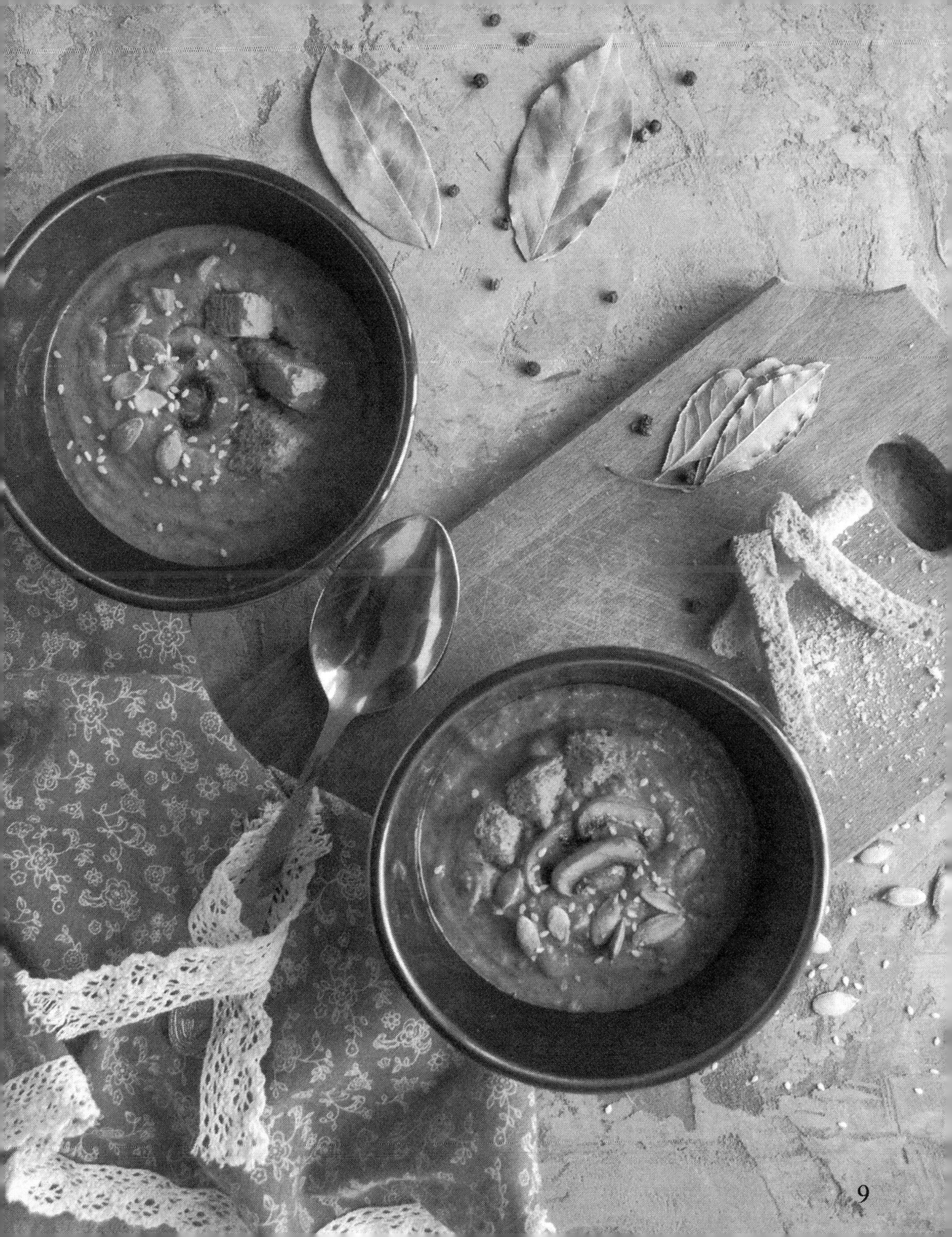

HOW TO KNOW WHEN YOU ARE IN KETOSIS

Whether you have taken any tests to discover your ketosis status, your body will exhibit physical signs to prompt you. You may have a loss of appetite, increased thirst, have bad breath, or notice a stronger urine smell. These are all clues from your body.

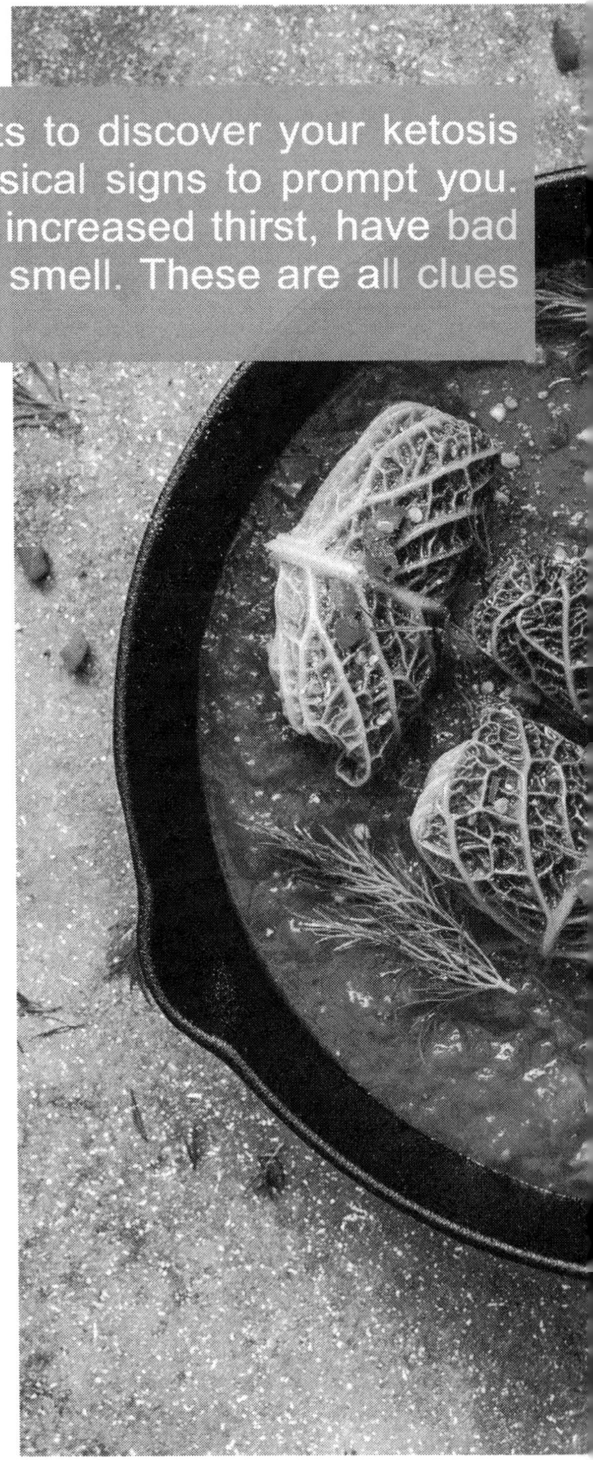

Ketosis and Your Sleep Patterns

After you have a good night of sleep, your body is in ketosis; since you have been in a fasted state for 8 hours or more, you are on the way to burning ketones. If you are new to high-fat and low-carb dieting, the optimal fat-burning state takes time. Your body has depended on bringing in carbs and glucose; it will not readily give up carbs and start to crave saturated fats.

The restless night is also a normal side effect. Vitamin supplements can sometimes remedy the problem that can be caused by a lowered insulin and serotonin level. For a quick fix, try one-half of a tablespoon of fruit spread and a square of chocolate.

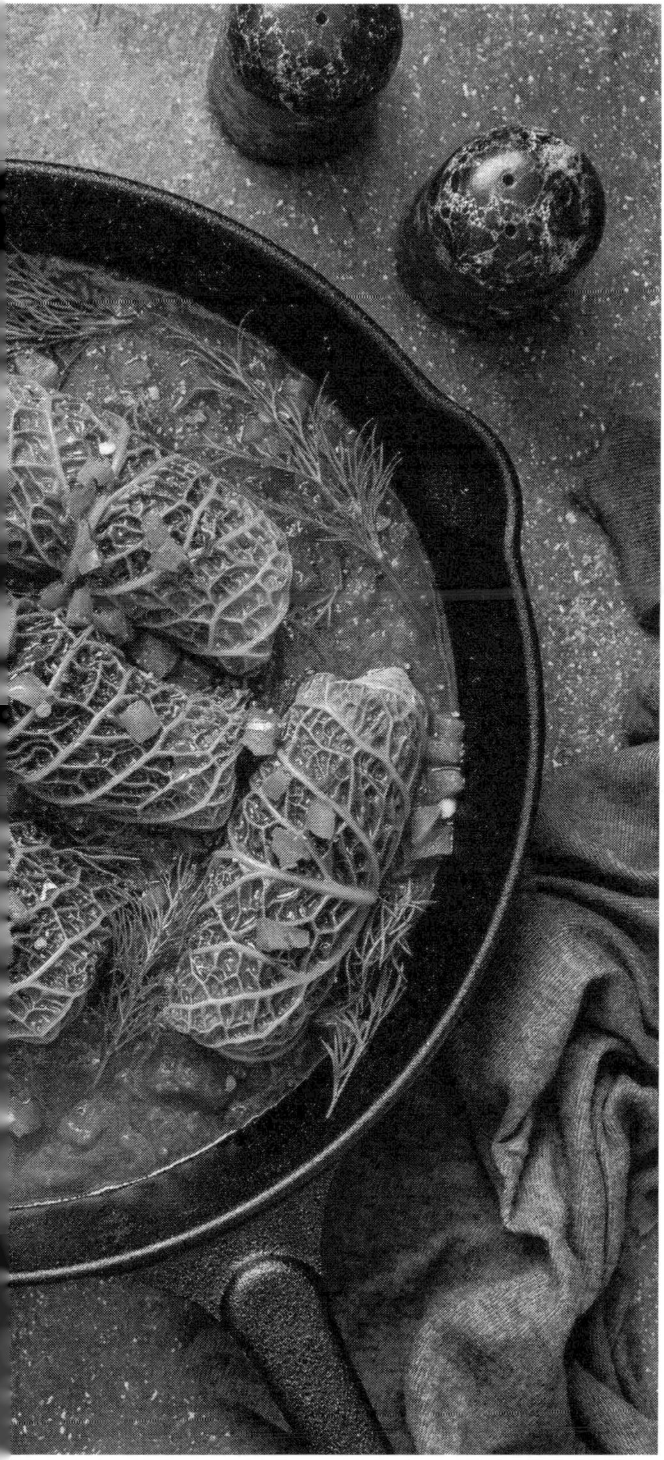

Bad Breath Happens

You may notice a metallic or fruity taste with an odor similar to nail polish remover. This is the by-product of acetoacetic acid (acetone), which is an obvious indication. You may also experience a drier mouth. These changes are normal as a side effect as your body processes these high-fat foods.

Once you are accustomed to the Ketogenic dieting techniques, the bad breath symptoms will pass. If you are socializing, try a diet soda or a no-sugar drink. Sugar-free gum is also a quick fix. Always check the nutrition labels for carbohydrate facts; you may be surprised. These are not allowed on the Keto diet because they reduce ketones. Therefore, only use it temporarily. If you are at home, just grab the toothbrush.

Lowered Appetite

When you reduce your carbs and proteins, you will be increasing your fat intake. The reduced appetite comes from the multitude of fibrous veggies, fats, and satiating nutrients provided in the new diet.

The "full" factor is a huge benefit to the Ketogenic plan. It will give you one less thing to worry about—being hungry.

Thirst is increased

Fluid retention is increased when you are consuming carbohydrates.

Once the carbs are flushed away, water weight is lost. You counterbalance by increasing the water intake since you are probably dehydrated.

The Keto diet calls for one to have more water intake because you are storing carbs. If you are dehydrated, your body can use the stored carbs to restore hydration.

When you're in ketosis, the carbs are removed, and your body doesn't have the water reserves. If you have tried other diets, you might have been dehydrated, but the higher carbohydrate counts stopped you from being thirsty.

Thus, the Keto state is a diuretic state, so drink plenty of water daily.

Digestive Issues

With the sudden change in diet, it's expected you may have problems including constipation or diarrhea when you first start the Keto diet. Individuals are different, and variation may rely on the foods you decide to eat to increase your fiber intake using various vegetables.

You may experience issues because your fiber intake may be too high in comparison to your previous diet. Try reducing certain "new" foods until the transitional phase of Keto is concluded. It should clear up with time.

You may be lacking beneficial bacteria. Try consuming fermented foods to increase your probiotics and aid digestion. You can benefit from B vitamins, omega-3 fatty acids, and beneficial enzymes as well.

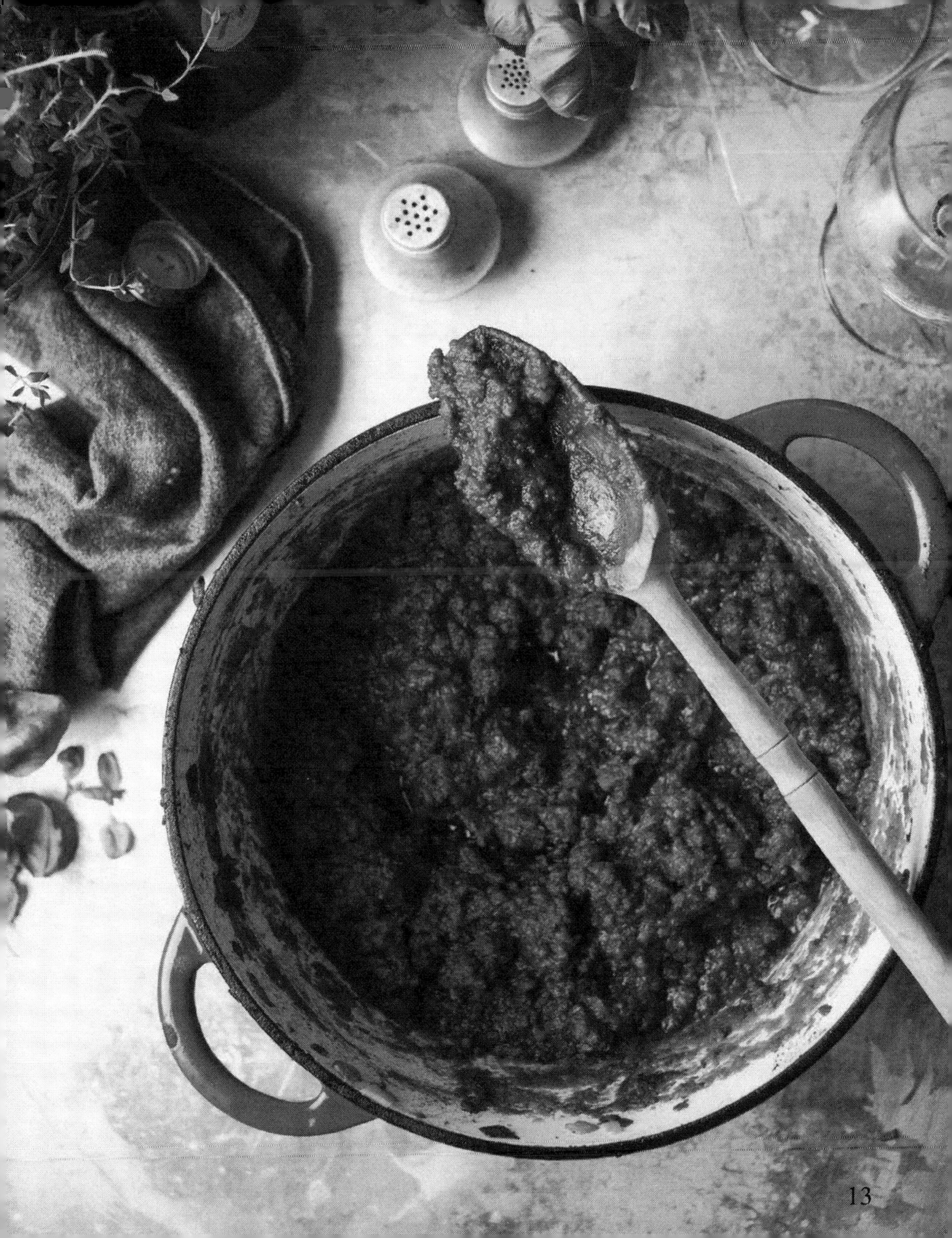

BENEFITS OF KETO DIET

The list of health benefits secured from a Keto Diet will never be ending. Nevertheless, for your convenience, a few of the more significant health benefits that you can gain from a Keto Diet will be explained.

Epilepsy

Since the Ketogenic diet is a diet that features high fat, low carbohydrate, and controlled consumption of protein, it causes the body to use fat as the primary energy source of energy. In a lot of epileptic cases, switching to a Ketogenic diet has resulted in a lowered incidence of seizures. Exercise care and supervision when children are following the diet.

Reversing Type 2 Diabetes

This is one of the benefits of being on a Ketogenic diet. There are many success stories about this diet, which research has proven is a result of lowering the number of carbohydrates that you consume, and as a result, your blood sugar level is brought to natural homeostasis. It is important to note that carb stimulates the body system to discharge the hormone called insulin. So, when carb intake is lowered, the body does not release more insulin to control the blood sugar, which will, in turn, increase the burning of fat that has been stored in the body. How then does this work in reversing Type 2 diabetes? The answer to the question is simple. The fundamental problem faced by people with diabetes is a high amount of blood sugar that comes primarily from carb intake. Once a person is on a Ketogenic diet, since they eat a fewer amount of carbs, the body can easily control the amount of blood sugar, which has the capacity of reversing Type 2 diabetes.

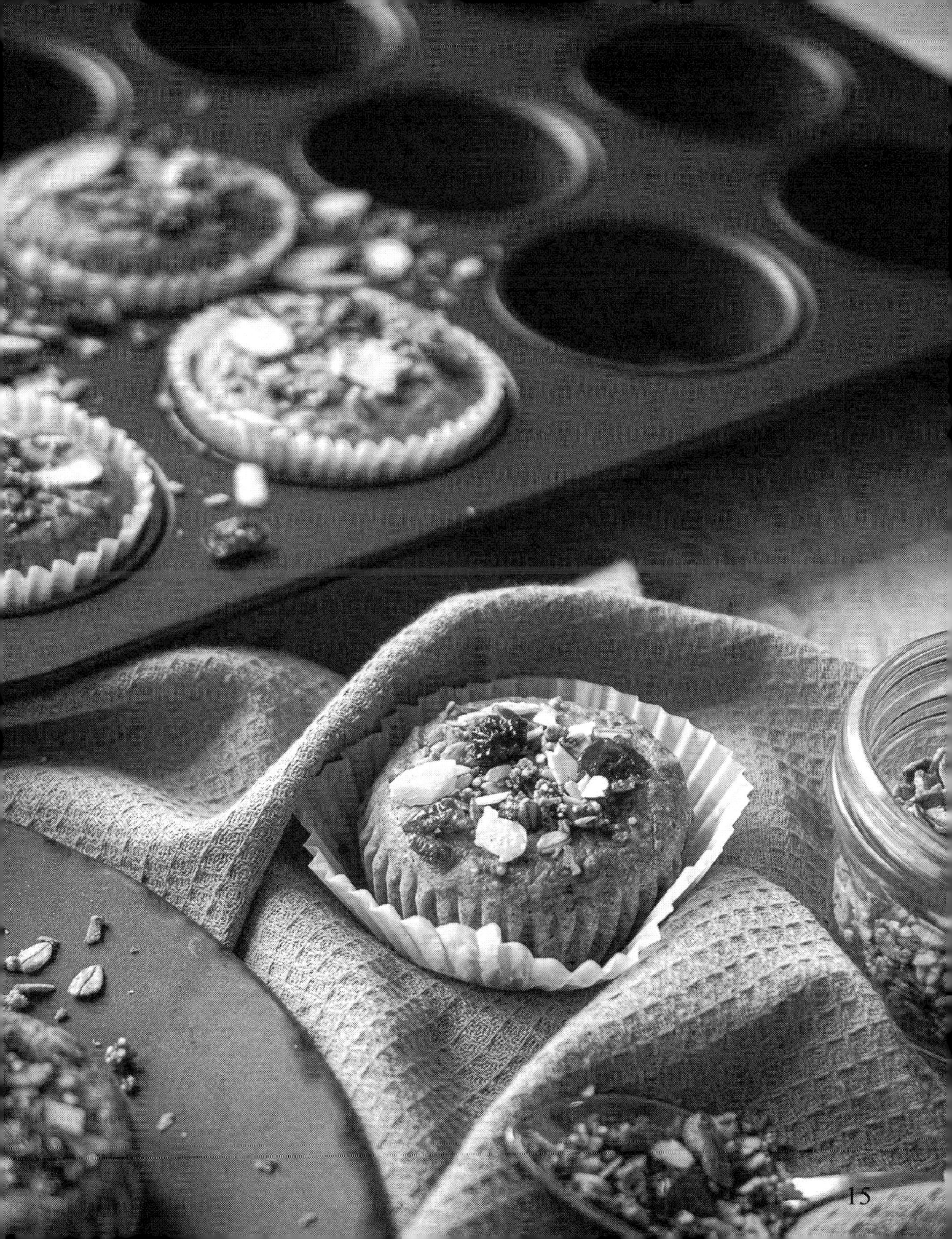

Effective Mental Agility

When ketosis mode is fully activated, there is a constant supply of ketones to the brain. Remember that when the body is not in ketosis mode and carb is steadily fed into the body system, the brain makes use of carb as a fuel source, and many are of the opinion that to increase mental agility and focus, more carbs need to be consumed. On the contrary, when you are fully in ketosis, your body registers a huge change in fuel consumption, meaning it burns more fat rather than the conventional carbs, resulting in fat in your body are broken down into ketone bodies. Other organs in the body can make use of fat. However, the brain makes use of ketones broken down from fat. During ketosis, there is usually an increase in the flow of ketone bodies to the brain, giving it a more effective mental agility and focus.

Acne Reduction

It has been reported with a colossal success that many people who have acne problems when on low carb diets like the Ketogenic diet, their acne is drastically reduced. When on a Ketogenic diet, the intake of carb is lowered. Where carbs are consumed, the body needs to produce the hormone called insulin to reduce the amount of blood sugar in the bloodstream. Acne is mostly caused and driven by insulin. It is the cornerstone of acne. Besides acting as the primary agent that motivate skin cells to manufacture sebum (an oily secretion secreted by the sebaceous gland for lubricating the hair and skin and protects against bacteria) and keratin (a fibrous insoluble protein that is the primary structural element in hair and nail), it heightens the secretion of many other hormones that causes acne. What does this all mean? When you are on a low carb diet like the Ketogenic diet, the flow of insulin to lower the amount of blood sugar in your bloodstream is not necessarily needed since your body does not require that. Insulin, being one of the leading causes of acne, will be curtailed since you do not consume many carbs that will summon its presence in your bloodstream. When there is no sugar to reduce in the blood, your insulin will not be used as often.

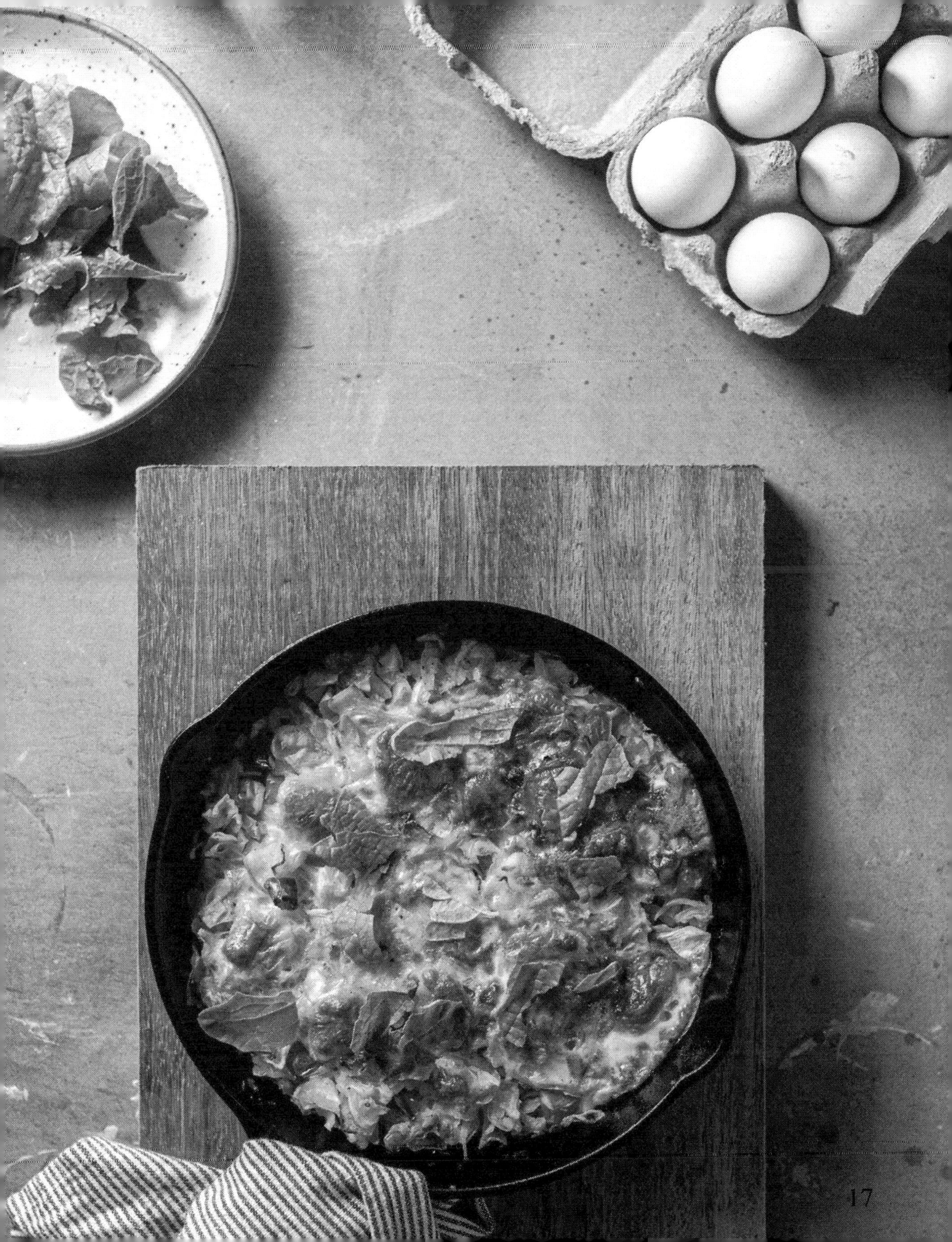

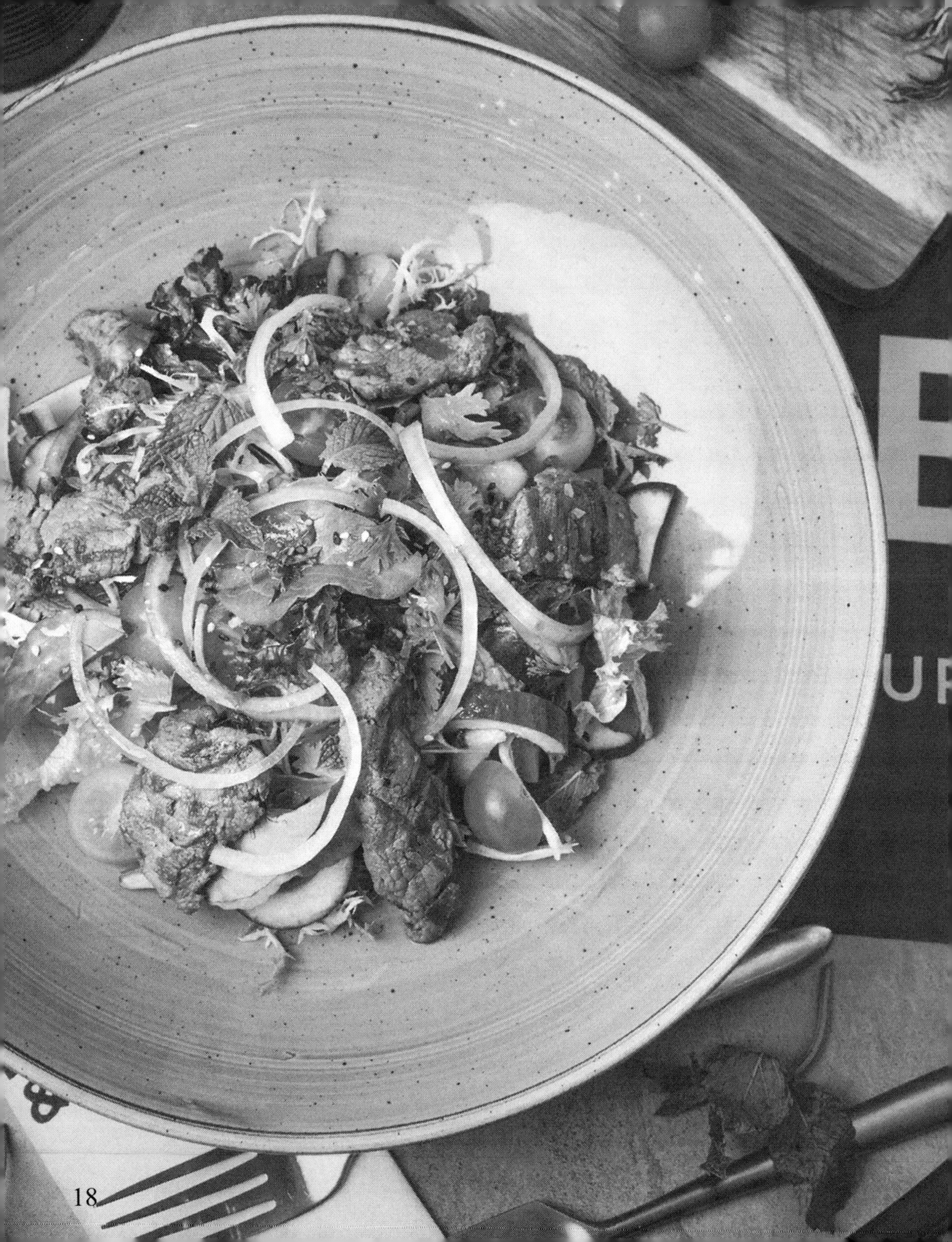

Weight Loss

What happens during ketosis? Your body shifts from burning carbs as fuel into burning fat, which results in tremendous weight loss. As you dive deeper into the sea of ketosis, your body burns fat resulting in weight loss. Instead of other types of diets, which many have been using for weight loss without success, with a Ketogenic diet, you lose body fat and weight quickly.

Enhanced Stamina

While practicing the Ketogenic diet, your physical stamina and endurance will be improved since you will have access to the storage of fat that your body has reserved. At a time of intense exercise, your stored carbs will melt away like the dissolving ice beaten down upon by summer light. On the other hand, your fat storage can last longer than your carbs. When you are carb adapted, your fat stores are quickly depleted during a short time of intense exercise, and to refill; you must keep eating. However, when you are on a Ketogenic diet, most of the fuel that is available is fat, with more long-lasting effects than your regular carb stores. Your body and your brain are energized by your fat stores, making you last longer in exercise and have more stamina than someone who is relying on carbs for their strength and endurance.

Enhanced Performance

Since your body is experiencing a shift from what it is used to, it is possible that at the formative stage of the Ketogenic diet, you might experience some form of reduced performance. But will this remain for a long time? Certainly not. The benefits of going Ketogenic are more long term than short term. Today many athletes are going Ketogenic, and they have improved their performance, especially in long-distance running. As I have explained earlier, your fat stores last longer than your carb stores. Since fat stores last longer, an athlete can perform for a prolonged period without refueling with external energy.

Decreased Aging

With the Ketogenic diet, your body can and will look younger for longer. When you have entered ketosis, ketone bodies are produced. These bodies may decrease the aging process by blocking a group of enzymes known as histone deacetylases. The enzymes function to keep a couple of genes known as Forkhead box O3 and Metallothionein 2A turned off. These genes can empower other cells to resist oxidative stress. The good thing is that the ketone bodies produce when full-fledge ketosis has been entered can block Forkhead box O3 allowing the genes to be reactivated, which prevents oxidative stress because it is this oxidative stress that indirectly causes aging. Besides, the Ketogenic diet reduces blood sugar levels. It is important to know that when sugar levels are reduced, glycation and the production of enhanced glycation by-product materials made from high blood sugar heightens tissue damage, diabetes, and aging. Finally, the Ketogenic diet is a catalyst that reduces triglycerides, which are known for causing a lot of terminal diseases.

Alzheimer's disease

This is a mental disorder that causes dementia because of the progressive degradation of the brain. One of the features of this disease is a decreasing ability to metabolize glucose. Whenever the mind is unable to metabolize glucose, it can have a lot of adverse effects on the brain. However, with ketone bodies, when a person is entirely into ketosis, the supply of ketones to the brain reduces the brain's over-dependence on glucose.

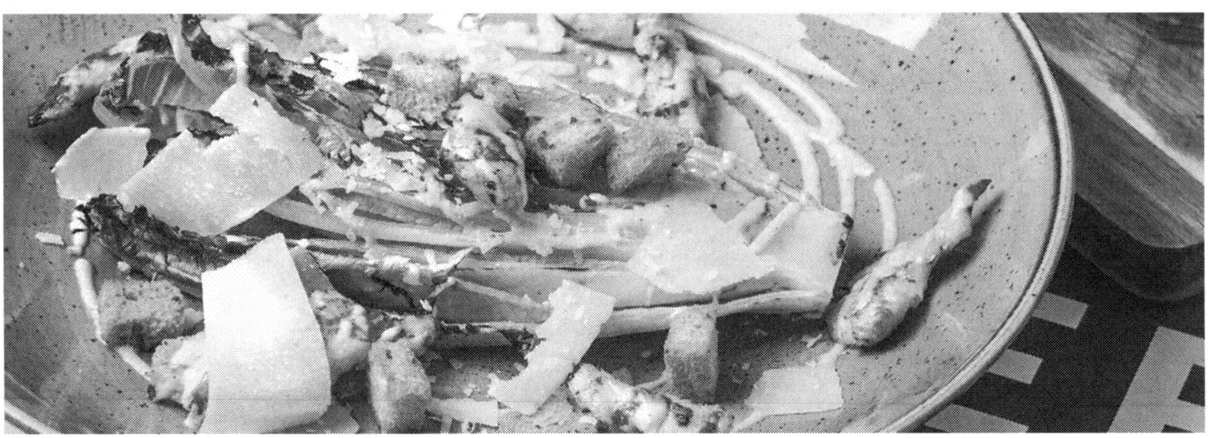

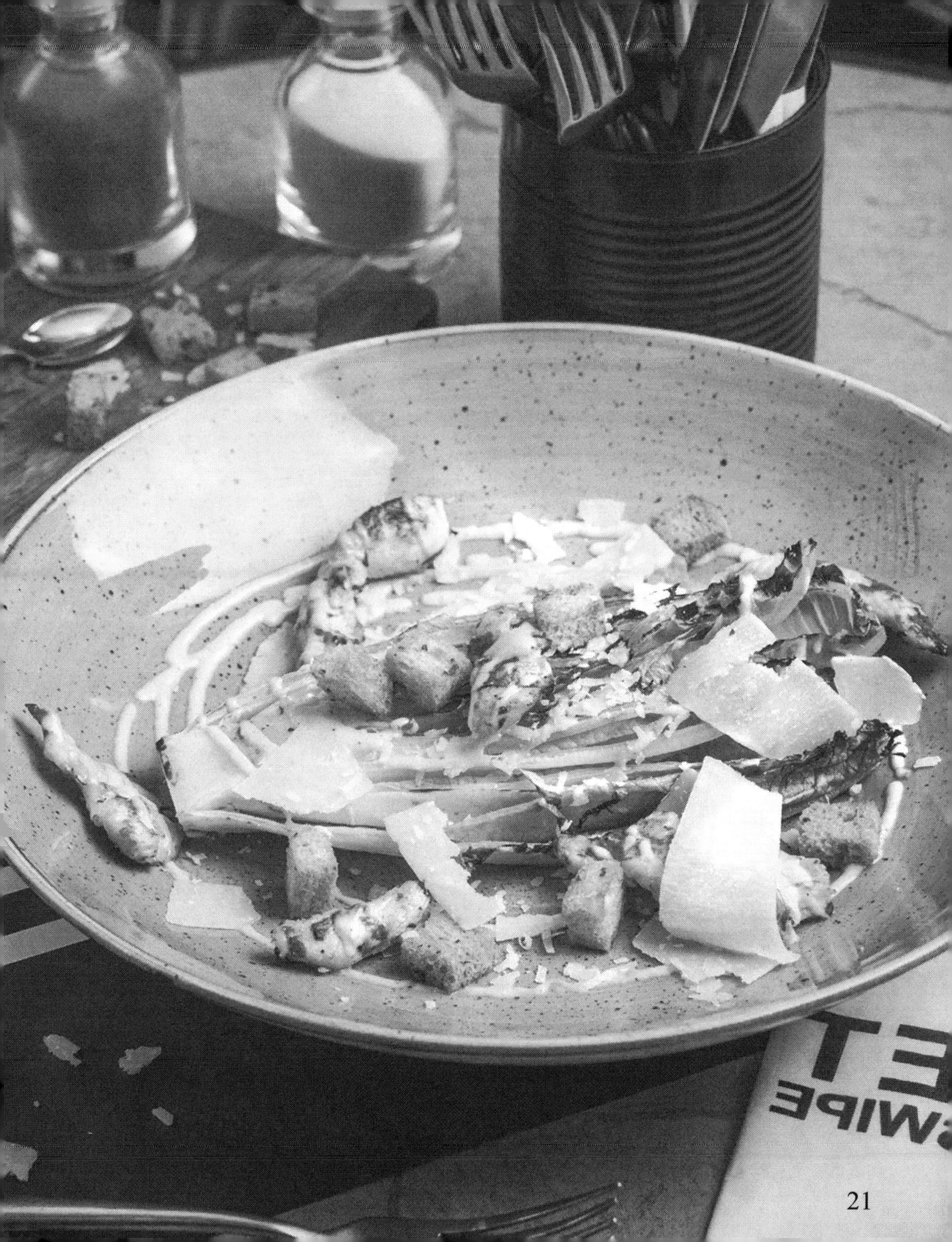

BREAKFAST RECIPES

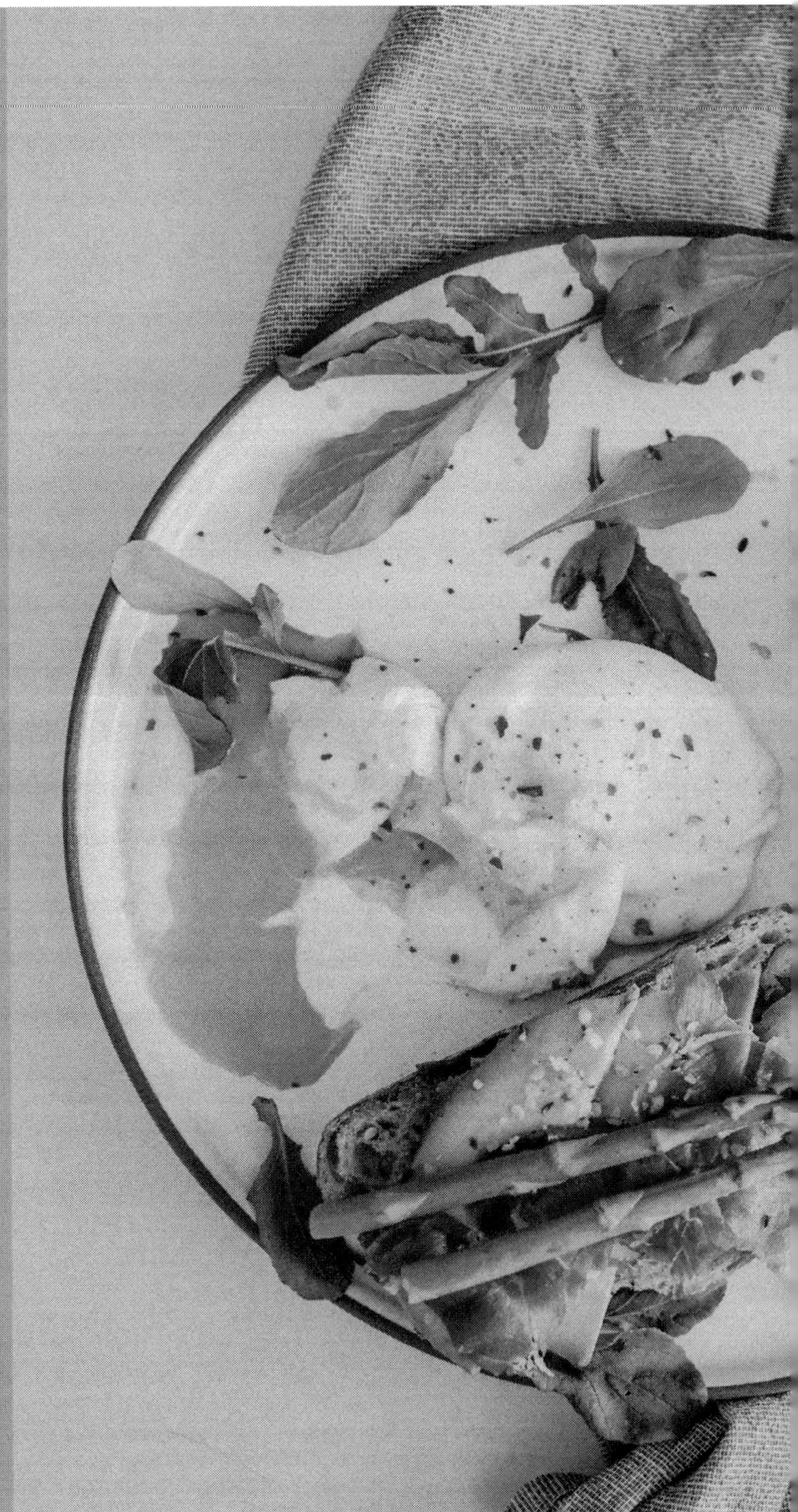

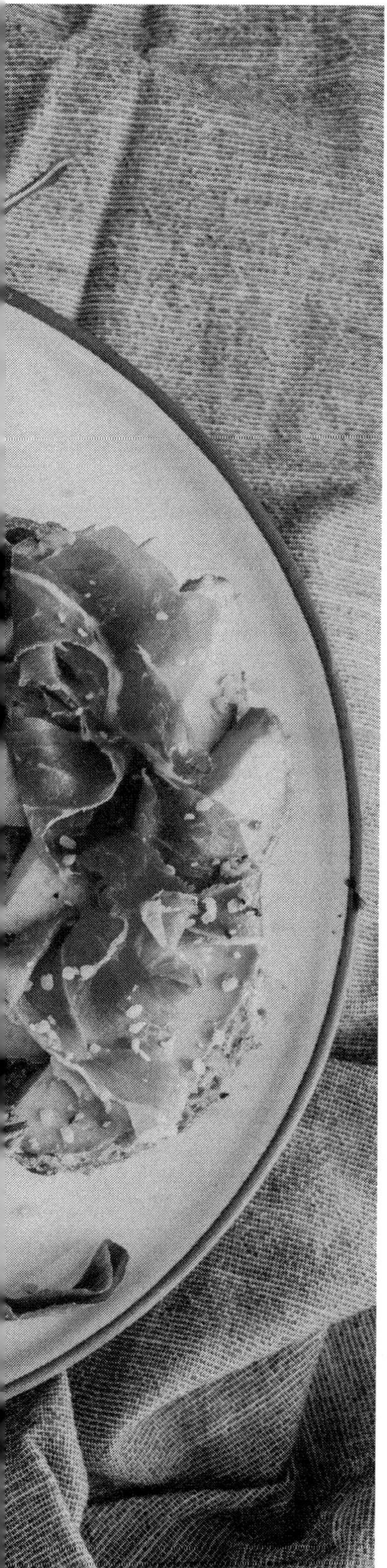

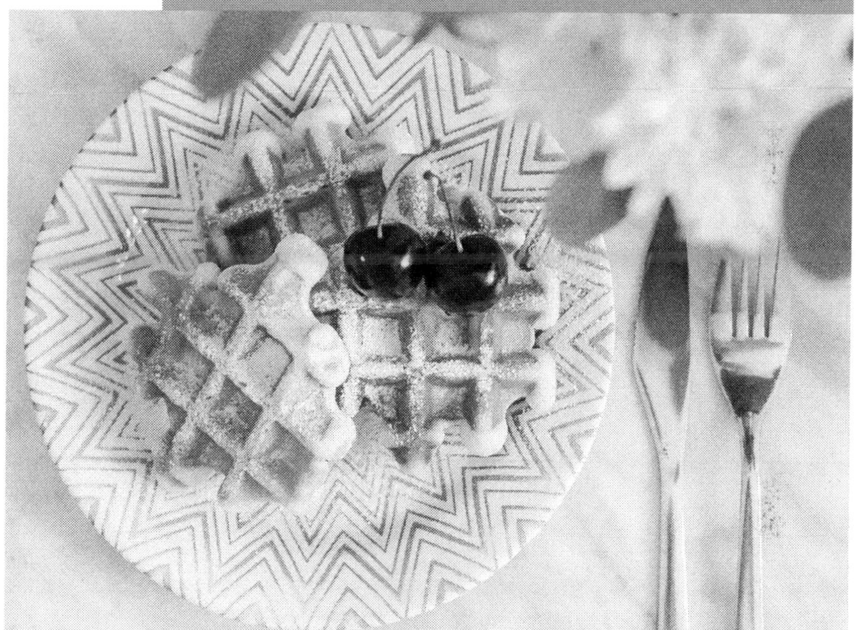

CHEDDAR SOUFFLES

Cooking Difficulty: 2/10	Cooking Time: 27 minutes	Servings: 8

INGREDIENTS

- 2 c. cheddar cheese
- ¾ c. heavy cream
- ¼ tsp. cayenne pepper
- ½ tsp. xanthan gum
- ½ tsp. pepper
- 1 tsp. ground mustard
- 1 tsp. salt
- ½ c. almond flour
- salt
- ¼ tsp. tartar cream
- 6 eggs
- ¼ c. chopped chives

STEP 1

Allow the oven to heat up to 350 degrees F. Take out a bowl and mix all the ingredients besides the eggs and cream of tartar together.

STEP 2

Separate the egg whites and yolks and add the yolks in with the first mixture. Beat the egg whites and cream of tartar until you get stiff peaks to form.

STEP 3

Take this mixture and add it into the other mixture. When done, pour into the ramekins and place in the oven.

STEP 4

After 25 minutes, these are done, and you can serve or store.

NUTRITIONAL INFORMATION

288 Calories, 21g Fats, 3g Net Carbs, and 14g Protein

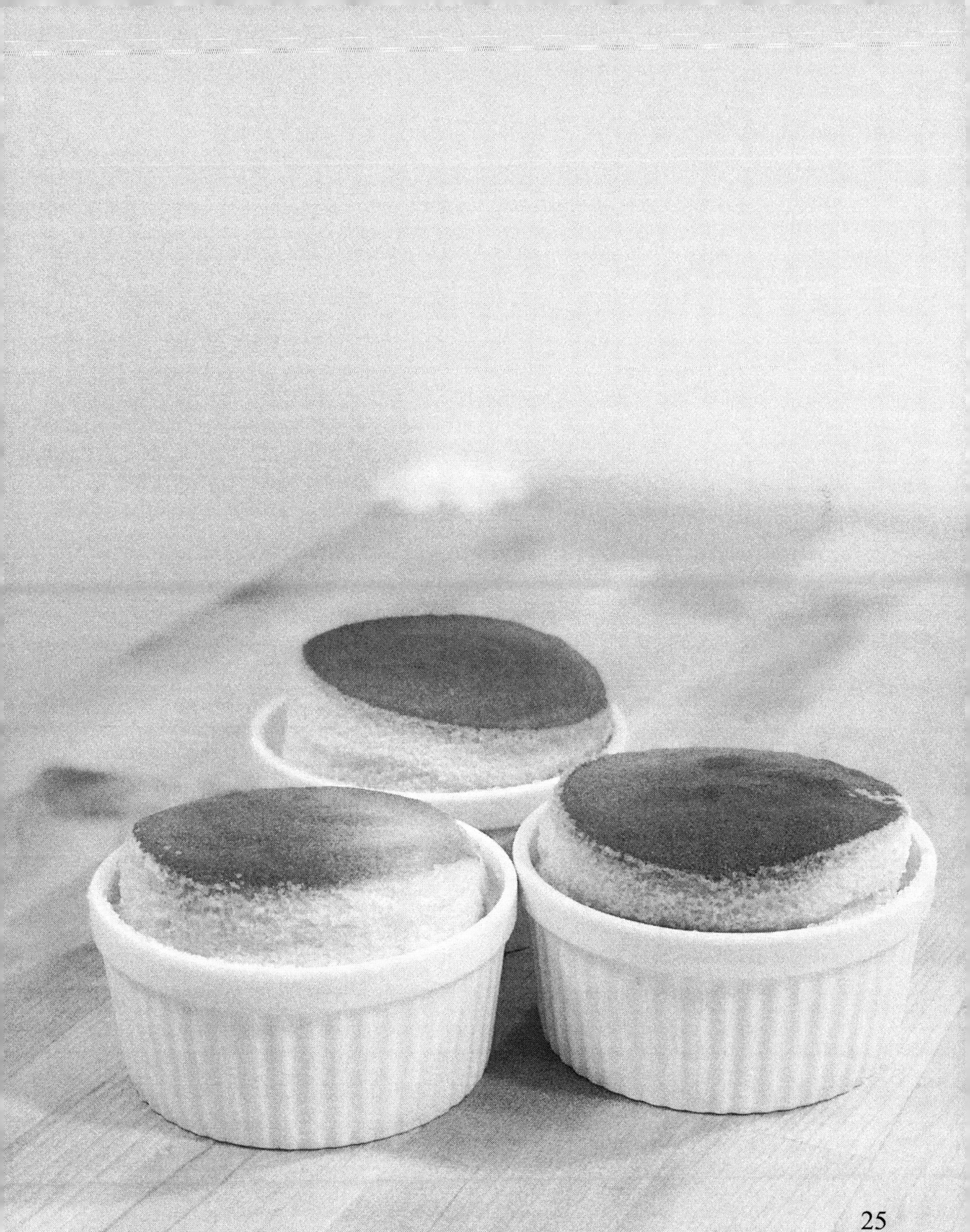

PARMESAN EGGS

Cooking Difficulty: 2/10	Cooking Time: 17 minutes	Servings: 1

INGREDIENTS

- 2 tbsps. Parmesan cheese, fresh and grated
- 1 tbsp. whipping cream
- 1 tbsp. butter, melted
- 1 egg

STEP 1

Preheat the oven to 350 degrees F.

STEP 2

Grease the ramekin with the butter. Dust with 1 tablespoon of the Parmesan cheese.

STEP 3

Crack the egg into the ramekin and cover with the cream. Sprinkle the remaining cheese to the mixture; bake for about 10-15 minutes, or until the egg white is set. Serve hot inside the ramekin.

NUTRITIONAL INFORMATION

308 Calories, 27.2g Fats, 1.9g Net Carbs, 15.8g Protein

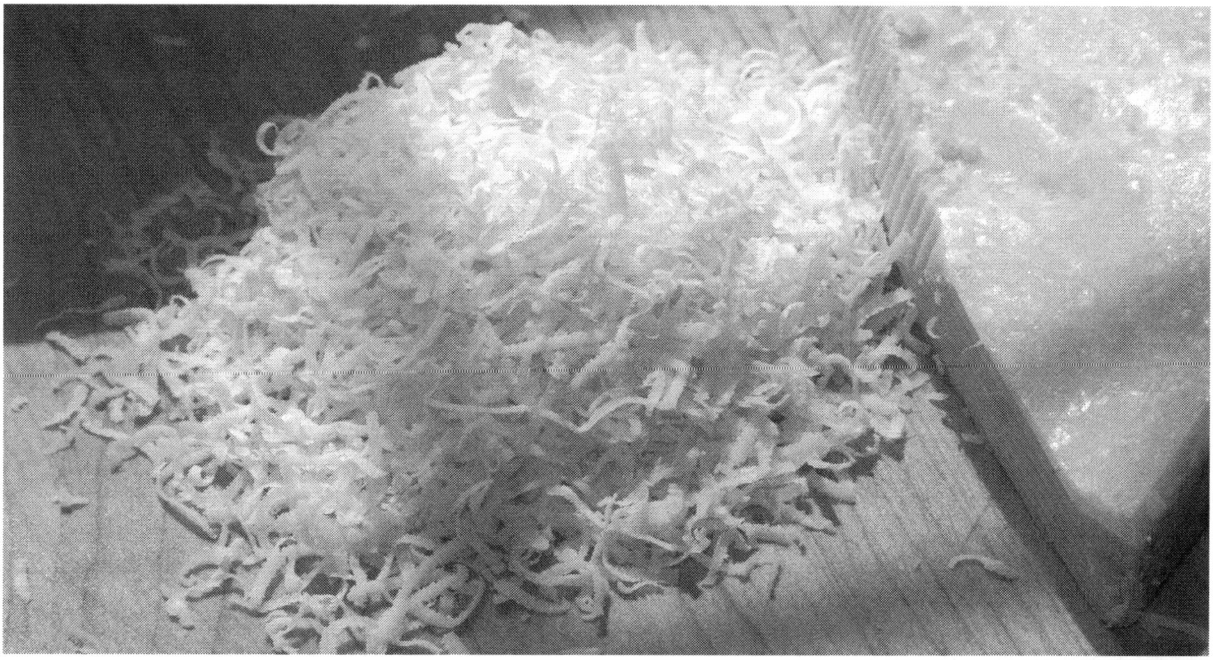

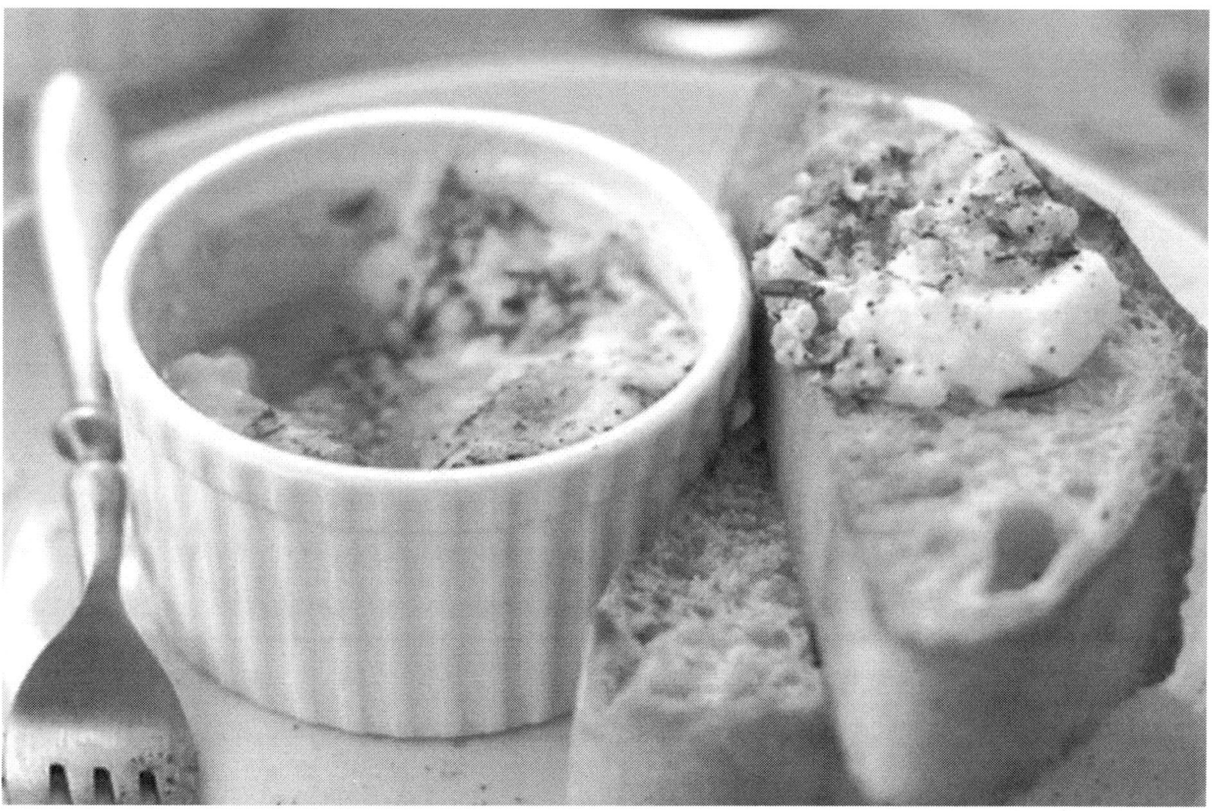

CHOCOLATE CHIP WAFFLES

Cooking Difficulty: 2/10	Cooking Time: 25 minutes	Servings: 2

INGREDIENTS

- ½ c. maple syrup
- 50g cacao nibs
- salt
- 2 tbsps. butter
- 2 separated eggs
- 2 scoop protein powder

STEP 1

Take out a bowl and beat the egg whites until soft peaks form. In a second bowl, mix the butter, protein powder, and egg yolks.

STEP 2

Now fold the egg whites into this mixture and add the cacao nibs and salt.

STEP 3

Pour the mixture into a waffle maker and let it cook until golden brown on both sides. Serve with maple syrup.

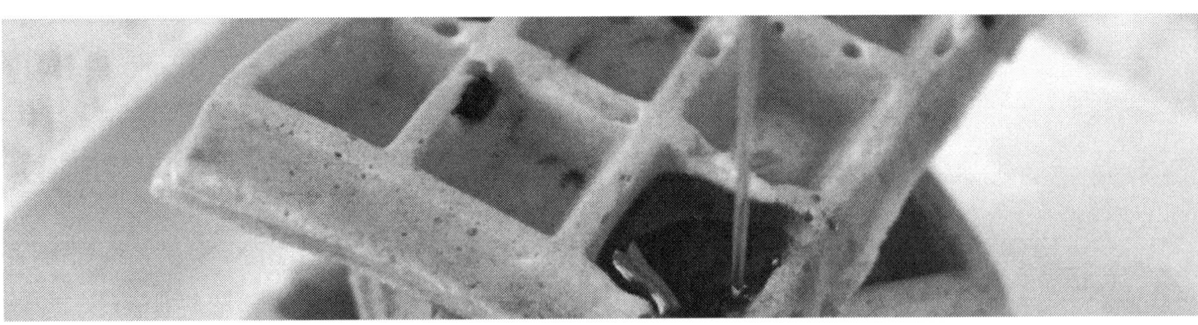

NUTRITIONAL INFORMATION

400 Calories, 26g Fats, 4.5g Net Carbs, 34g Protein

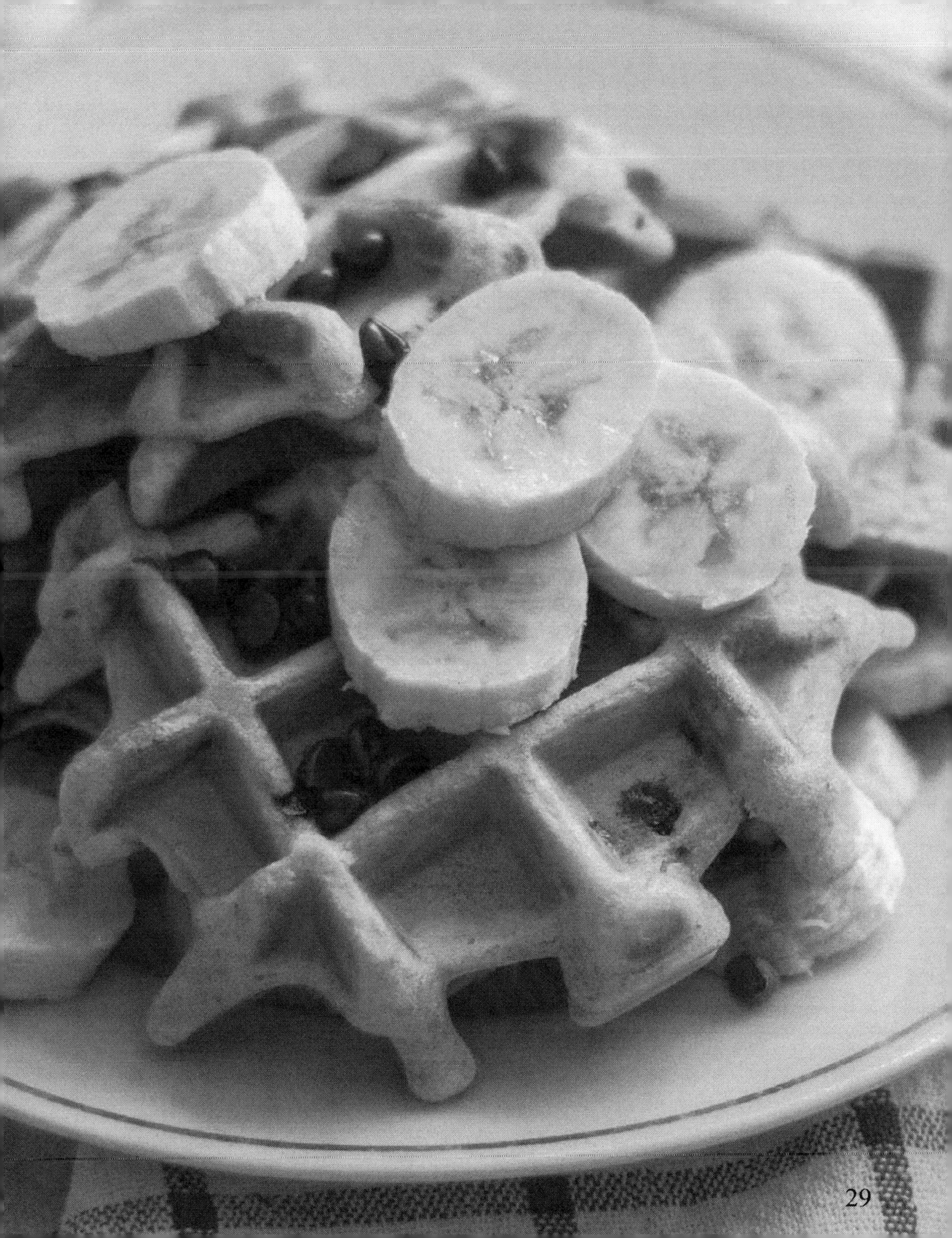

BLACKBERRY EGG BAKE

Cooking Difficulty: 2/10	Cooking Time: 17 minutes	Servings: 4

INGREDIENTS

- 1 tsp. chopped rosemary
- ½ tsp. orange zest
- salt
- ¼ tsp. vanilla
- 1 tsp. grated ginger
- 3 tbsps. coconut flour
- 1tbsp. butter
- 5 egg
- ½ c. blackberries

STEP 1

Allow the oven to heat up to 350 degrees F. Take out a blender and add all the ingredients inside to blend well.

STEP 2

Pour this into each muffin cup and then add the blackberries on top. Place into the oven to bake.

STEP 3

After 15 minutes, take the dish out and store!

NUTRITIONAL INFORMATION

144 Calories, 10g Fats, 2g Net Carbs, 8.5g Protein

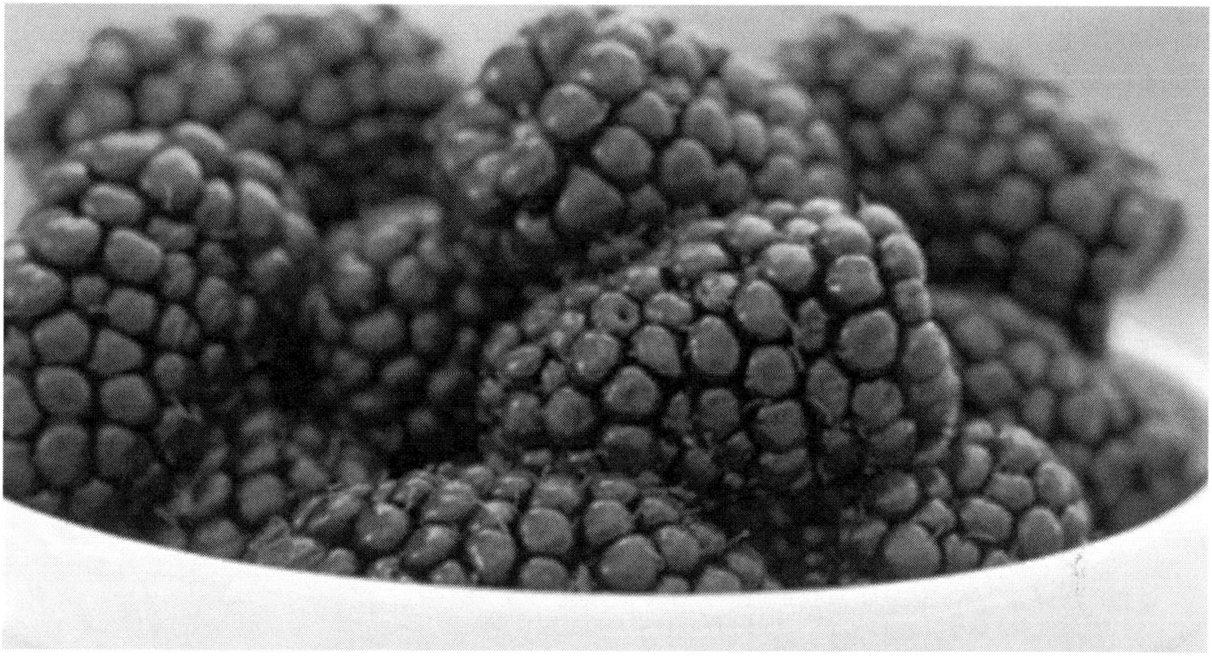

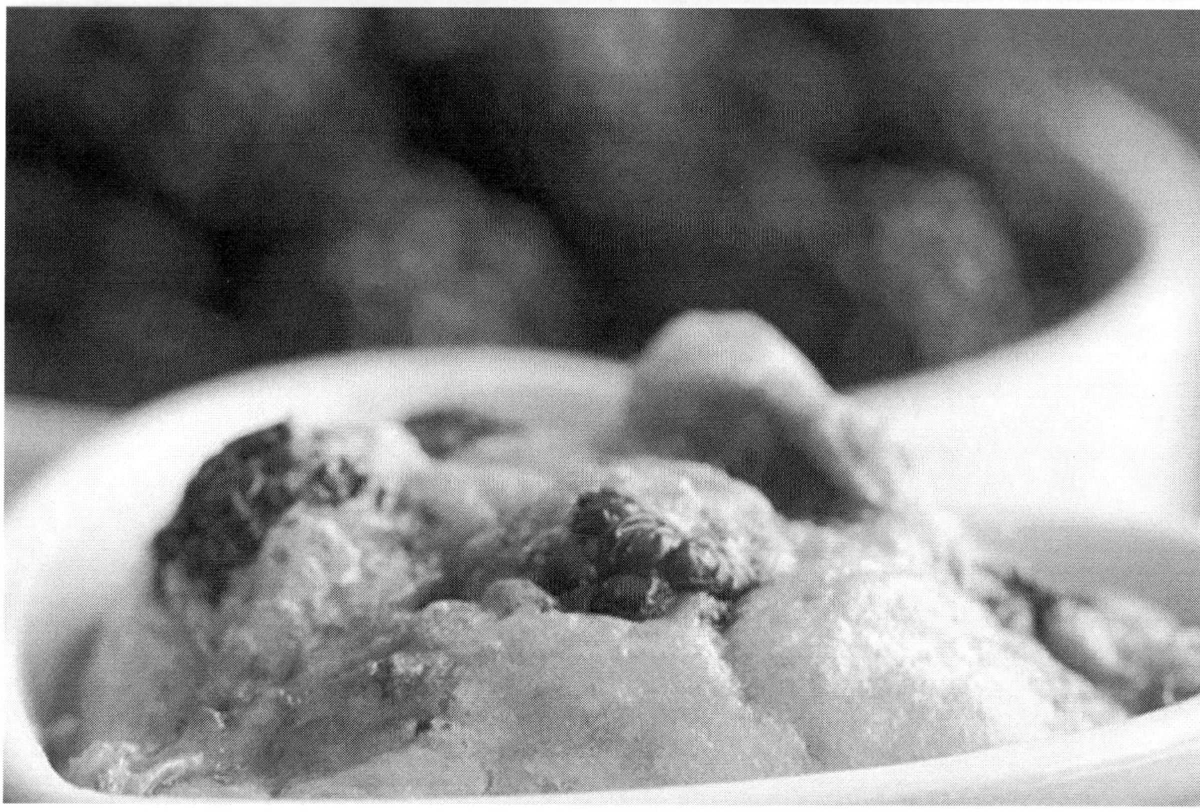

EASY SCOTCH EGGS

Cooking Difficulty: 3/10	Cooking Time: 30 minutes	Servings: 6

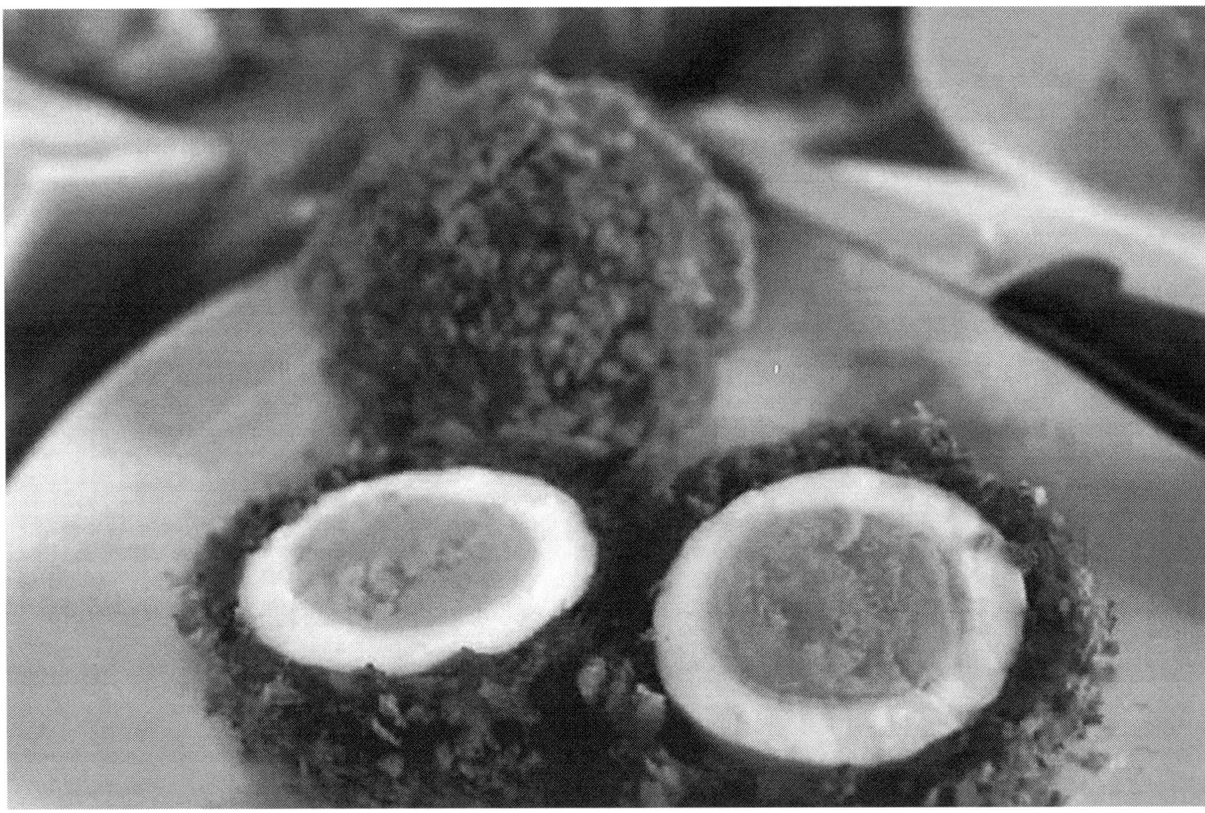

NUTRITIONAL INFORMATION

258 Calories, 21g Fats, 1g Net Carbs, and 17g Protein

INGREDIENTS

- 6 hardboiled eggs, peeled
- 1½ c. breakfast sausage
- 1½ tsps. garlic powder
- 1/3 tsp. sea salt
- ½ tsp. black pepper

STEP 1

Set the oven to 400 degrees F to preheat.

STEP 2

Spread a large sheet of baking paper on a clean, dry surface.

STEP 3

Place the breakfast sausage in a large bowl and add the salt, pepper, and garlic powder. Mix well with clean hands.

STEP 4

Divide the breakfast sausage mixture into 6 equal balls and arrange on the sheet of baking paper. Flatten the sausage balls out, then place a hardboiled egg on top. Wrap the egg with the sausage mixture.

STEP 5

Arrange the sausage-coated eggs on a dry baking sheet and bake in the preheated oven for 25 minutes.

STEP 6

Arrange the scotch eggs on a cooling rack and let sit for 5 minutes. Store in an airtight container and refrigerate for up to 4 days. Reheat before serving.

CHEESE AND SAUSAGE IN PORTOBELLO BURGERS

Cooking Difficulty: 3/10	Cooking Time: 17 minutes	Servings: 4

INGREDIENTS

- 8 portobello mushroom caps
- 8 oz. American cheese
- ¼ c. breakfast sausage
- 4 tbsps. olive oil

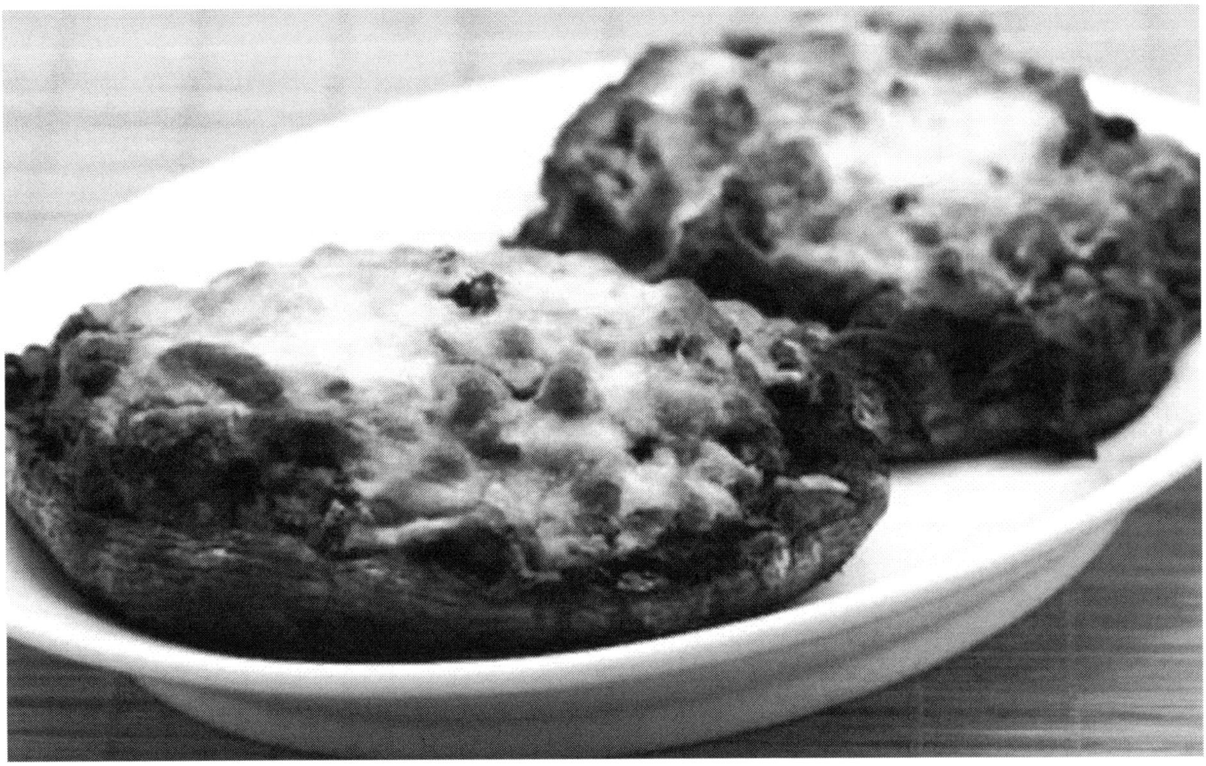

NUTRITIONAL INFORMATION

504 Calories, 41g Fats, 10g Net Carbs, 24g Protein

STEP 1
Rinse the mushroom caps thoroughly, removing and discarding the stems and gills. Blot dry with paper towels and set aside.

STEP 2
Place a large cast-iron skillet over medium flame and heat through. Once hot, add a quarter of the olive oil and swirl to coat.

STEP 3
Add two of the Portobello mushroom caps and cook for 5 minutes per side, or until browned all over. Transfer to a platter and repeat with the remaining mushroom caps. Set aside.

STEP 4
Divide the breakfast sausage into four patties.

STEP 5
Wipe the skillet clean and reheat over medium flame. Add half of the remaining olive oil and swirl to coat. Add two of the patties and cook for about 2 to 3 minutes per side, or until cooked through.

STEP 6
Add a slice of American cheese on each patty, then cover the pan and cook until the cheese is melted.

STEP 7
Slice the patties with the melted cheese into the mushroom caps. Repeat with the remaining patties and cheese slices until four patties have patties.

STEP 8
Cover the top of the mushroom caps with the other patties until you have four "burgers."

STEP 9
Wrap each "burger" in aluminum foil and refrigerate for up to 3 days, or freeze for up to 3 weeks. Reheat before serving.

SAVORY CHEDDAR PANCAKES

Cooking Difficulty: 3/10	Cooking Time: 18 minutes	Servings: 4

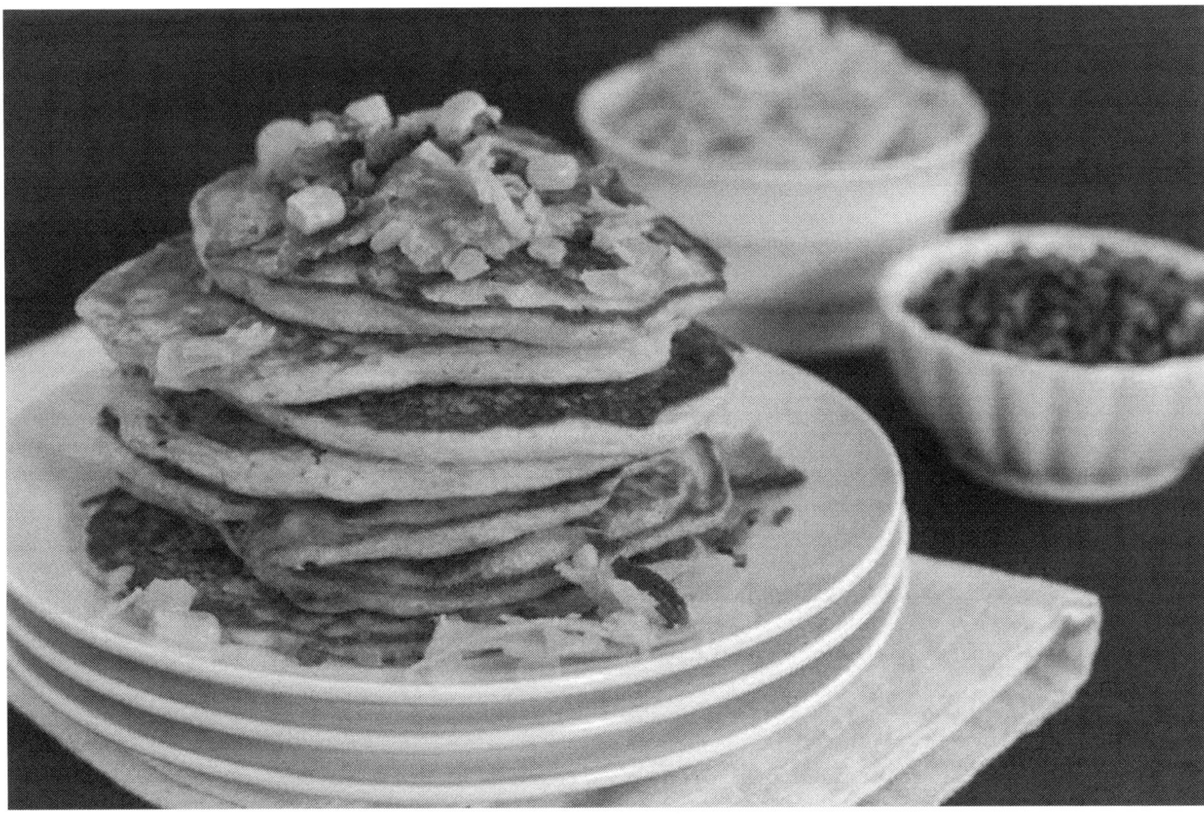

NUTRITIONAL INFORMATION

257 Calories, 24g Fats, 2g Net Carbs, and 11g Protein

INGREDIENTS

- 4 large egg whites
- 4 oz. grated cheddar cheese
- 2 c. almond meal
- 4 tbsps. olive oil
- 1 tbsp. chopped green onion
- 1 tsp. baking powder

STEP 1

Combine the almond meal, water, grated cheddar cheese, green onion, and garlic in a large bowl. Mix well and set aside.

STEP 2

Whisk the egg whites in a separate bowl together with the baking powder, then add the almond meal mixture. Beat everything well until smooth.

STEP 3

Place a pancake griddle or nonstick skillet over medium-high flame and heat through. Add a bit of olive oil and swirl to coat.

STEP 4

Once hot, ladle in an eighth of the batter into the hot skillet and cook for 1 minute per side, or until set.

STEP 5

Transfer to a platter, then repeats with the remaining batter. Place in an airtight container and refrigerate for up to 3 days. Reheat before serving.

BREAKFAST SQUARES

Cooking Difficulty: 2/10	Cooking Time: 38 minutes	Servings: 2

INGREDIENTS

- 8 oz. shredded mozzarella cheese
- 8 oz. shredded cheddar cheese
- large eggs
- sliced jalapeno peppers
- 4 tbsps. butter

STEP 1

Carefully mix the cheeses and eggs.

STEP 2

Butter the bottom of a skillet; add the pepper and the cheese mixture; Set oven to 350F, and bake for 35 minutes, then for 30 more minutes at 250 degrees F.

STEP 3

Serve.

NUTRITIONAL INFORMATION

782 Calories, 62.6g Fats, 4.4g Net Carbs, 51.6g Protein

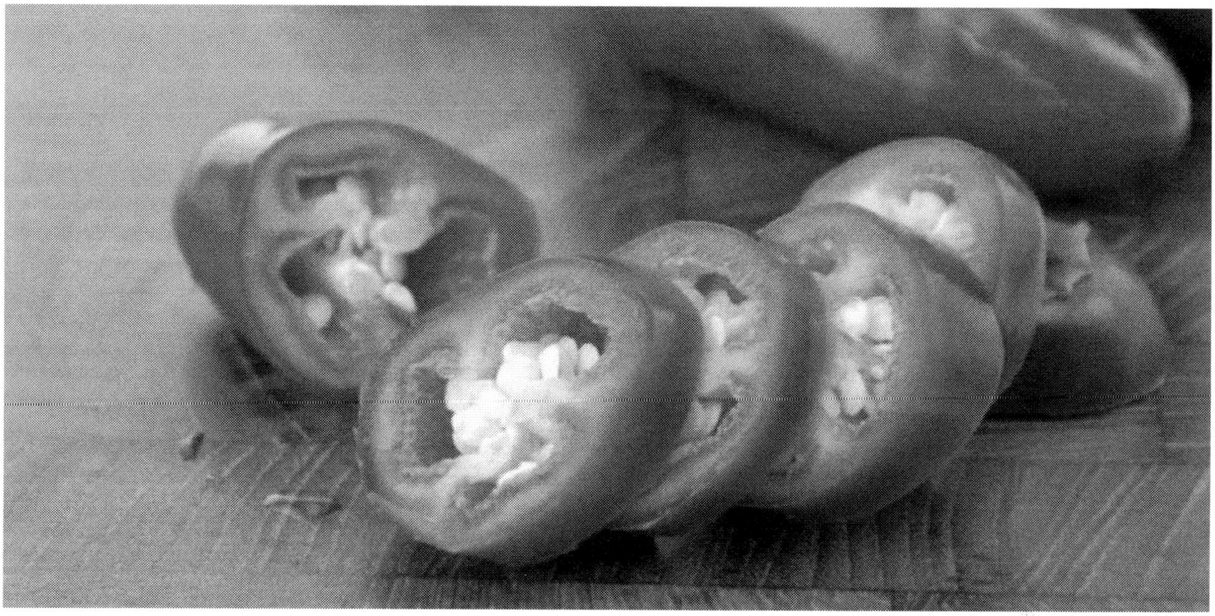

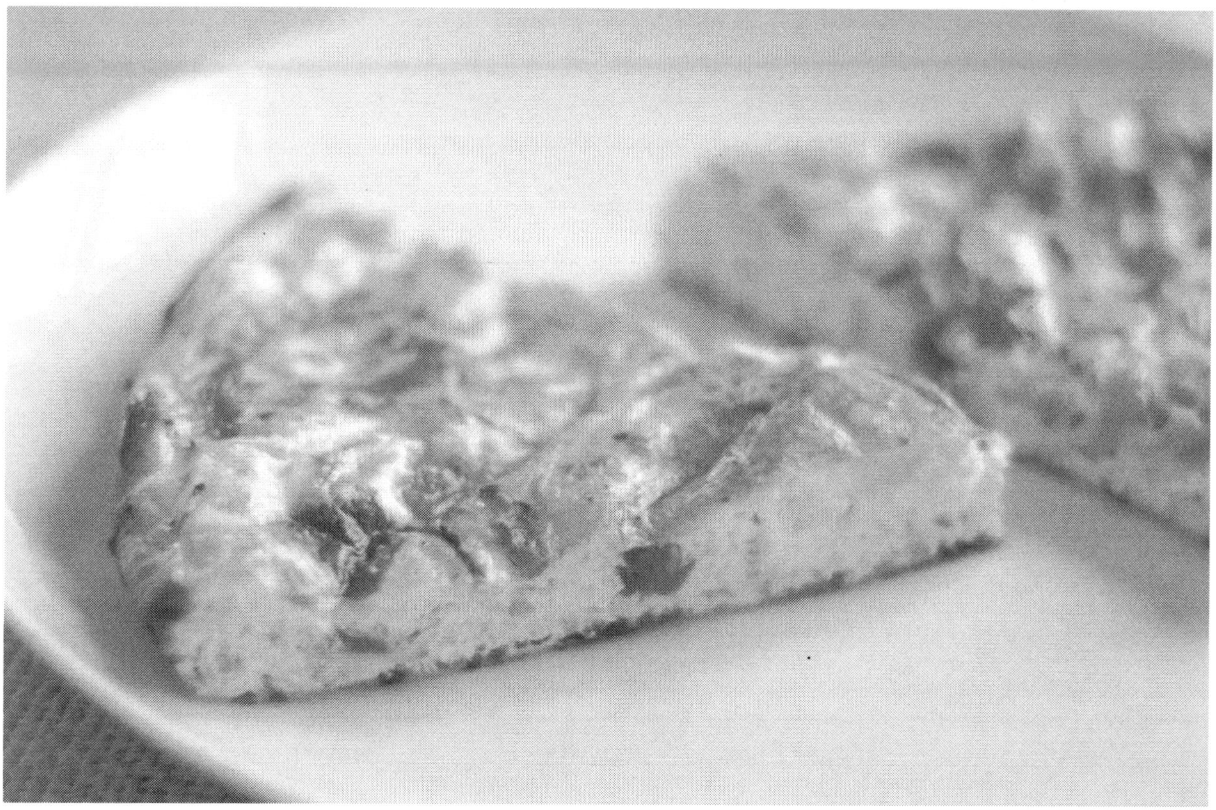

CAJUN TOFU SCRAMBLE

Cooking Difficulty: 2/10	Cooking Time: 9 minutes	Servings: 2

INGREDIENTS

- 14 ounces drained and cubed tofu
- ½ yellow onion
- 1 diced red bell pepper
- 1 diced zucchini
- 2 teaspoon cajun seasoning
- kale

STEP 1

Saute onions in a skillet until transparent.

STEP 2

Add tofu and seasonings.

STEP 3

Cook for five minutes.

STEP 4

Add vegetables and cook until tender, approximately eight minutes.

NUTRITIONAL INFORMATION

224 Calories, 12g Fats, 14g Net Carbs, 22g Protein

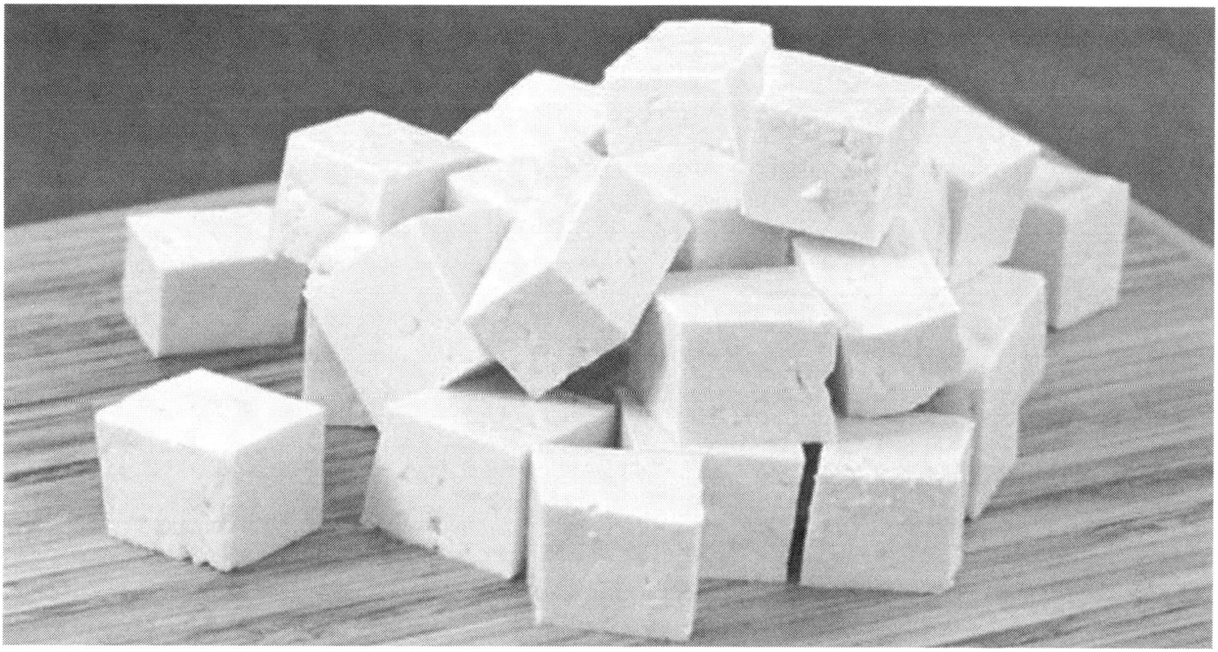

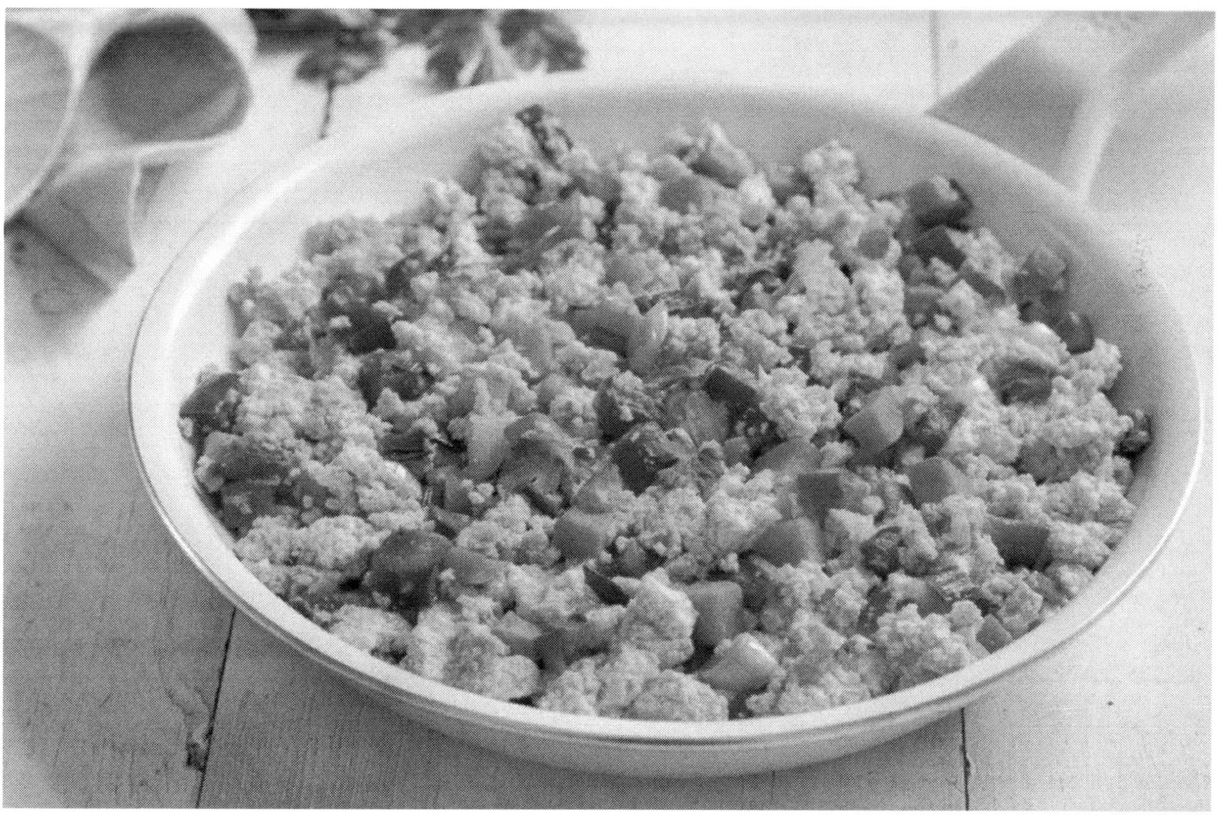

ALMOND BREAKFAST MUFFINS

Cooking Difficulty: 3/10	Cooking Time: 17 minutes	Servings: 4

INGREDIENTS

- 1¼ c. almond flour
- ½ tsp. sea salt
- ½ tsp. baking soda
- 3 large eggs
- ¼ c. almond slivers
- 3 tbsps. coconut oil
- 1 tbsp. coconut flakes
- 6 bacon strips
- 1 c. grated parmesan cheese
- 2 tsps. stevia
- 1 tsp. vanilla

STEP 1

In a mixing bowl, pre-sift the blanched almond flour to obtain the desired consistency. Add eggs and then vanilla; give about 30 strokes with a large spoon and add almond slivers, coconut flakes, stevia, and 2 tablespoons of coconut oil.

STEP 2

In a coconut oil greased cupcake pan, scoop about two tablespoons of batter and bake at 350 degrees F for about 15 minutes.

STEP 3

Garnish with crumbled bacon just as they come out of the stove.

NUTRITIONAL INFORMATION

221 Calories, 17.7g Fat, 2.9g Carbs, 13.4g Protein

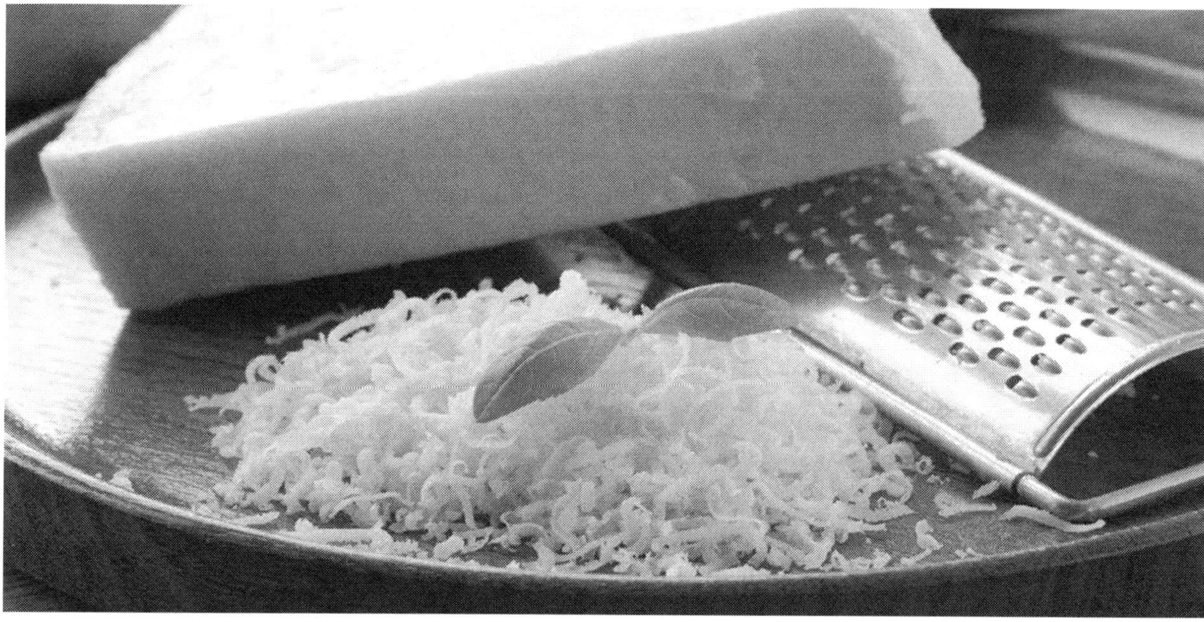

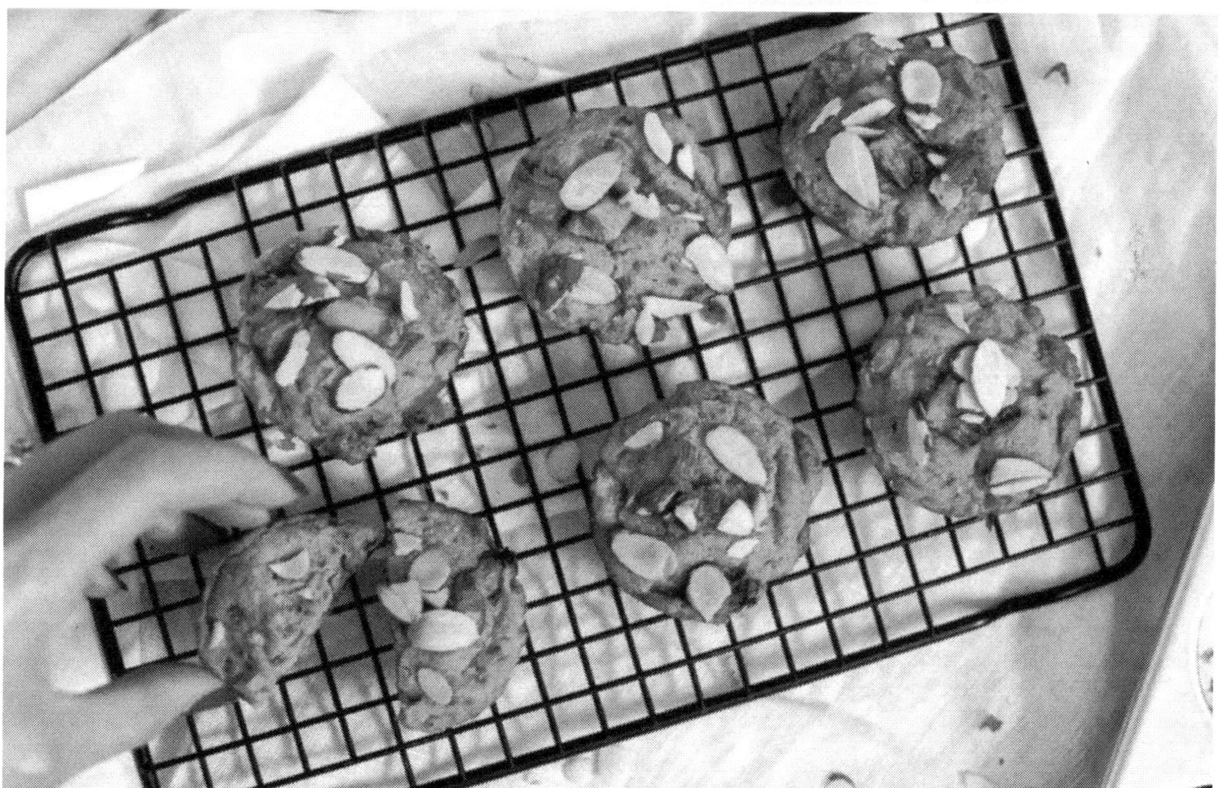

CHIA CINNAMON VANILLA GRANOLA

Cooking Difficulty: 3/10	Cooking Time: 29 minutes	Servings: 6

INGREDIENTS

- 56g whey protein powder
- 1 c. macadamia nuts
- ¼ c. water
- 4 tbsps. flaxseed meal
- 4 tbsps. whole chia seeds
- 4 tbsps. coconut oil, melted
- 3 tbsps. water
- 4 tsps. stevia
- 2 tsps. cinnamon
- 1 tsp. pure vanilla extract
- ¼ tsp. fine sea salt

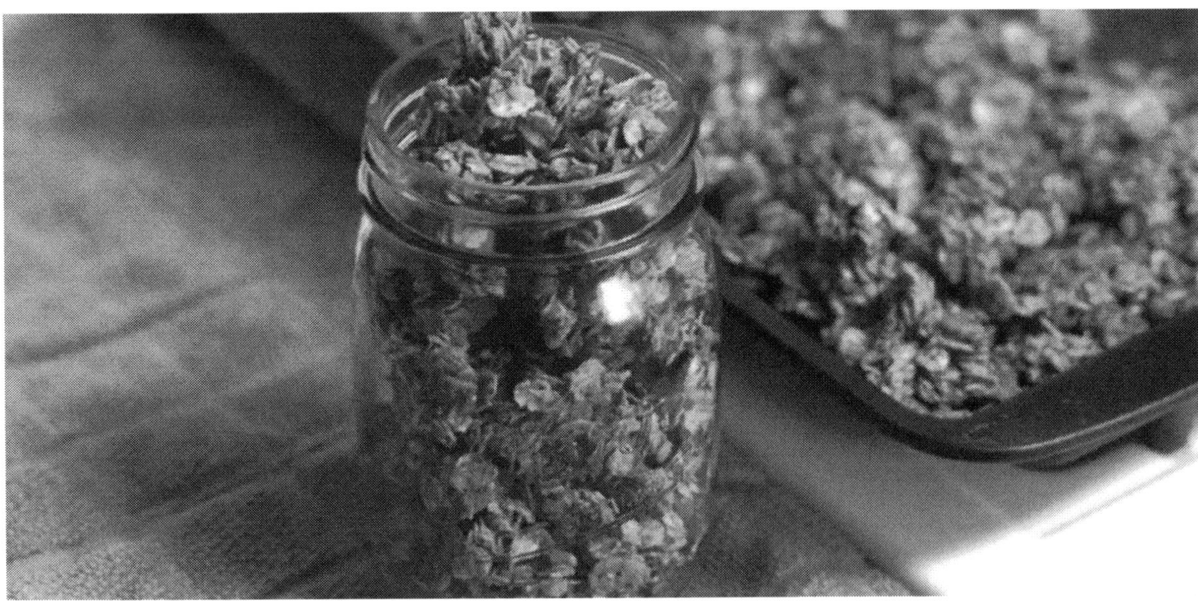

NUTRITIONAL INFORMATION

336 Calories, 31g Fats, 11g Net Carbs, and 9g Protein

STEP 1

Set the oven to 350 degrees F to preheat. Line a baking sheet with baking paper and set it aside.

STEP 2

Mix together the vanilla extract, water, and chia seeds in a large bowl. Set aside for 5 minutes, or until the mixture becomes gelatinous.

STEP 3

Pour the macadamia nuts into a food processor, then add the flaxseed meal, protein powder, stevia, salt, and cinnamon. Pulse until the mixture is fine and the nuts are grounded.

STEP 4

Pour the gelatinous chia seed mixture into the food processor, then add about 1 ½ tablespoon of water and the coconut oil. Blend until the mixture is smooth. Set aside.

STEP 5

Using a tablespoon, transfer the mixture onto the prepared baking sheet. Then, transfer to the oven and bake for 15 minutes.

STEP 6

Once baked, remove from the oven and break into small pieces. Spread out on the pan.

STEP 7

Bake for an additional 10 minutes, or until the granola is dry and golden brown. Set on a cooling rack and allow to cool completely.

STEP 8

Transfer to an airtight container and store for up to 1 week in the refrigerator. Best served with warm milk.

EASY BREAKFAST TACOS

Cooking Difficulty: 3/10	Cooking Time: 11 minutes	Servings: 2

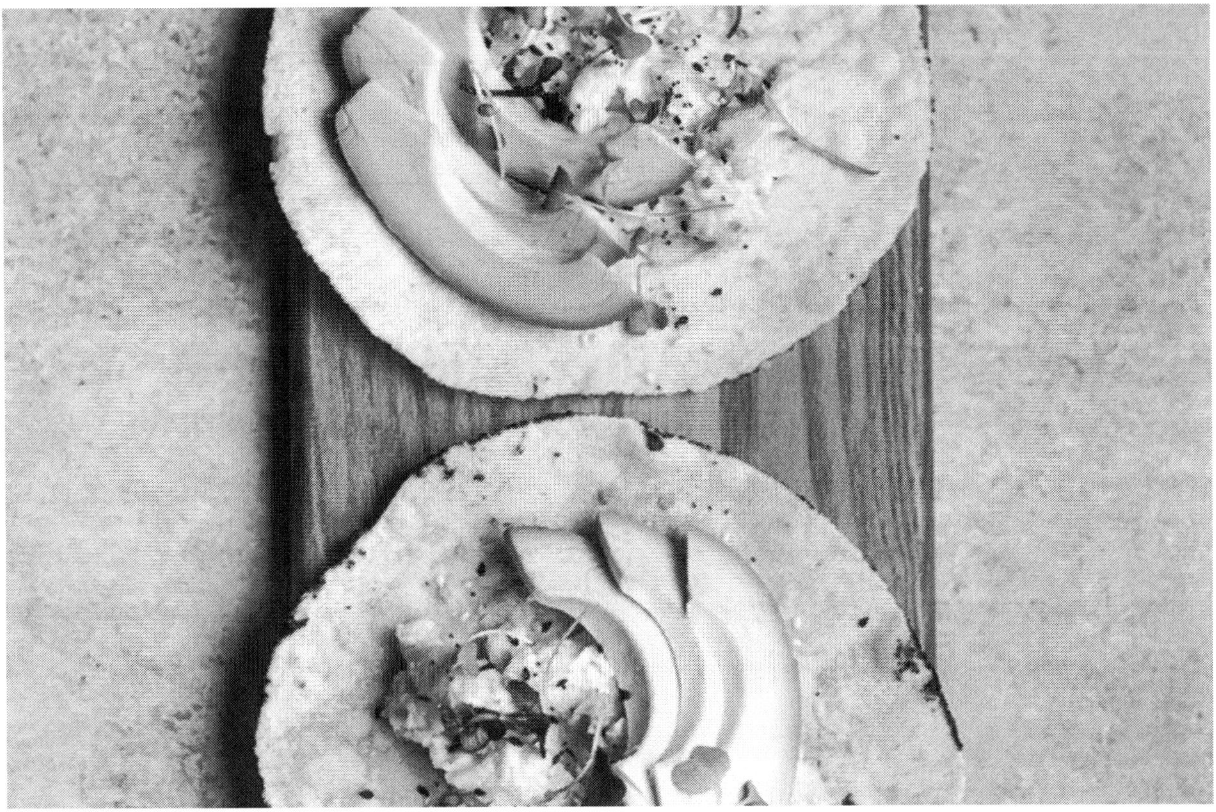

NUTRITIONAL INFORMATION

289 Calories, 27g Fats, 6g Net Carbs, 7g Protein

INGREDIENTS

- 2 low carb tortillas
- 4 large eggs
- ½ sliced avocado
- 2 tbsps. mayonnaise
- 1 tbsp. butter
- 4 fresh cilantro sprigs
- tabasco sauce
- sea salt
- black pepper

STEP 1

Whisk the eggs in a bowl until smooth. Set aside.

STEP 2

Place a nonstick skillet over medium flame and heat through. Once hot, add the butter and swirl to coat.

STEP 3

Add the egg and tilt until the eggs are spread out. Cook until done, then transfer to a bowl. Set aside.

STEP 4

Warm the tortillas over a low flame, then place on a platter and spread the mayonnaise on one side of each tortilla.

STEP 5

Divide the egg between the two tortillas, then add the sliced avocado, and cilantro. Season with salt and pepper, then add the pepper sauce. Roll up the tortillas and serve.

STEP 6

To store, add lime juice all over the avocado first before placing in the tortilla. Wrap tightly in aluminum foil and store in the freezer for up to 1 day. Reheat in a toaster oven before serving.

CINNAMON COCONUT PORRIDGE

Cooking Difficulty: 2/10	Cooking Time: 12 minutes	Servings: 4

INGREDIENTS

- 2 c. water
- 1 c. 36 percent heavy cream
- ½ c. unsweetened dried shredded coconut
- 2 tbsps. oat bran
- 2 tbsps. flaxseed meal
- 1 tbsp. butter
- 1½ tsps. stevia
- 1 tsp. cinnamon
- sea salt

STEP 1

Combine all the ingredients in a small pot and mix well until smooth.

STEP 2

Place the pot over a medium-low flame and bring to a slow boil. Once boiling, stir well and remove from the heat.

STEP 3

Divide into four equal servings and set aside for 10 minutes to thicken. Best served warm. Store in mason jars, seal tightly, and refrigerate for up to 2 days.

NUTRITIONAL INFORMATION

171 Calories, 16g Fats, 6g Net Carbs, 2g Protein

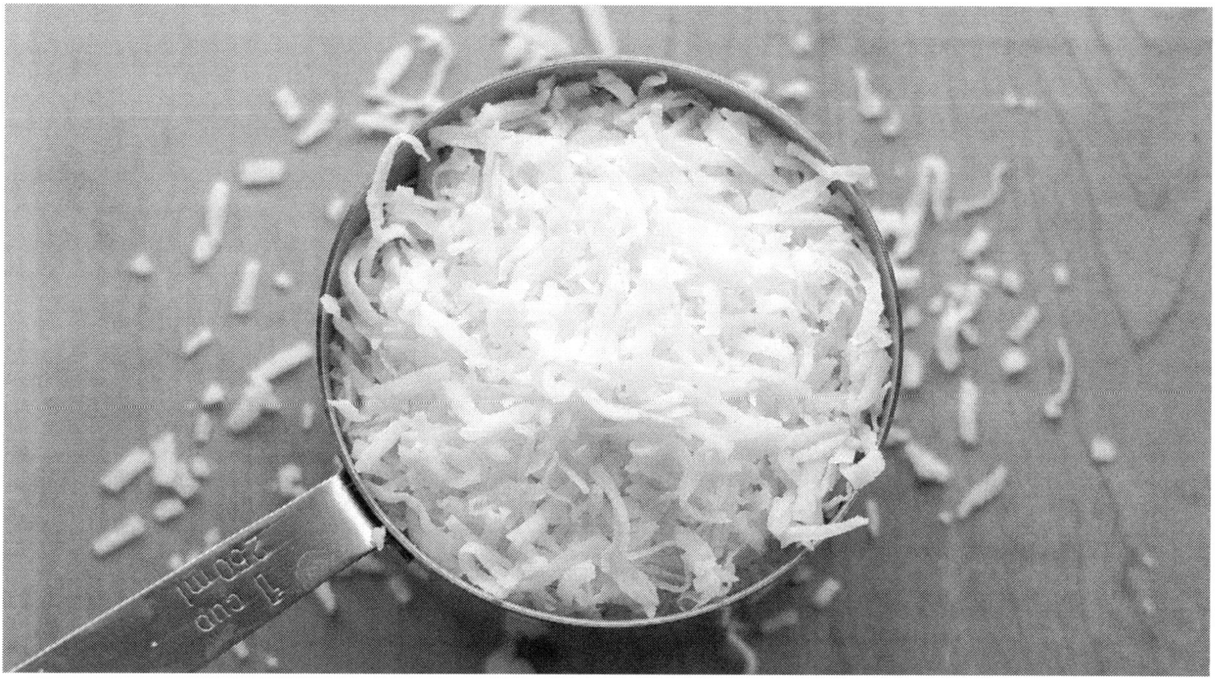
1 cup
250ml

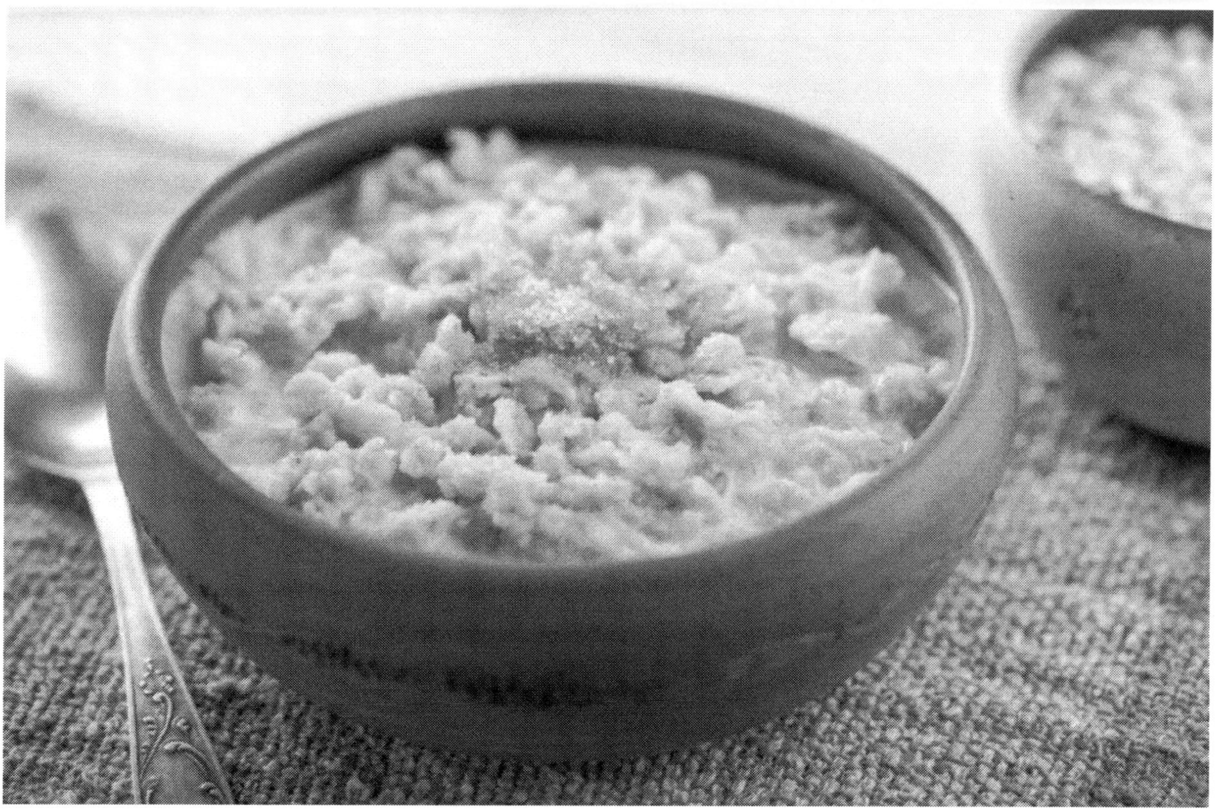

CHEESE KETO QUICHE

Cooking Difficulty: 4/10	Cooking Time: 110 minutes	Servings: 8

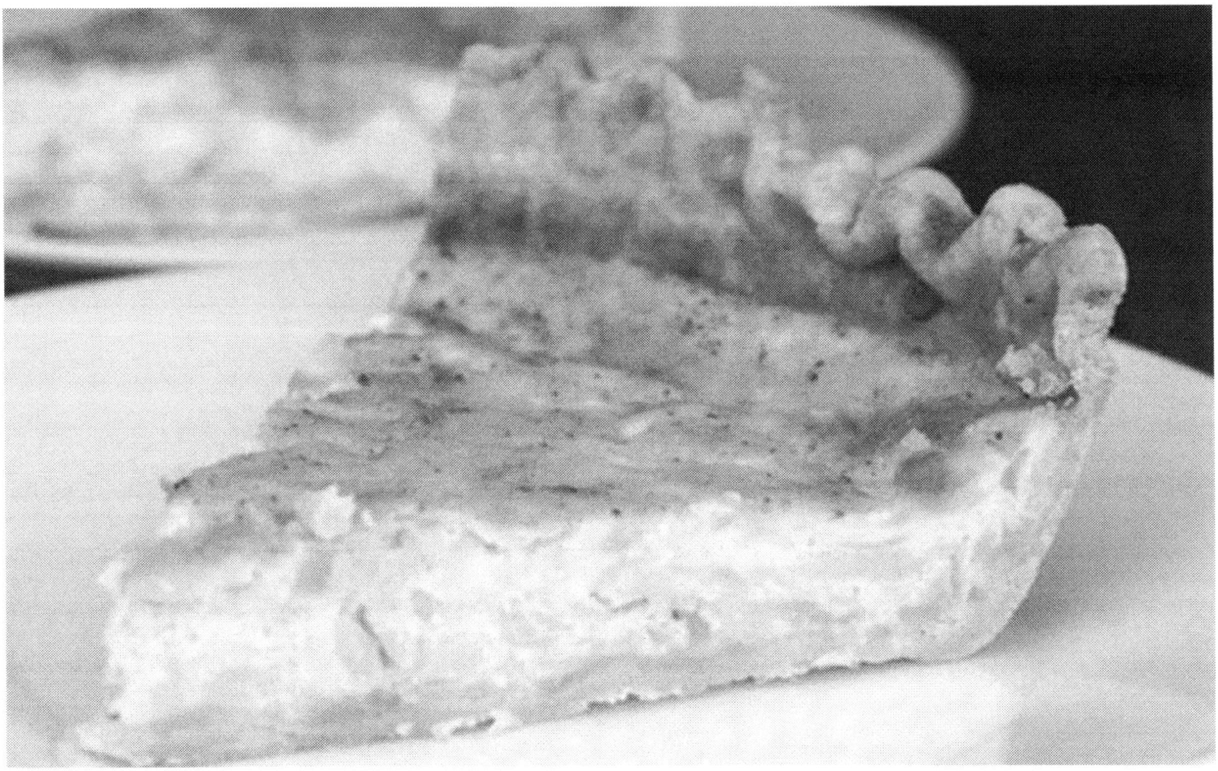

INGREDIENTS

for the crust:

- 2 large raw egg whites
- 1 c. almond flour
- 2/3 c. dry roasted macadamia nuts
- ¾ c. extra virgin olive oil
- ½ tsp. fine sea salt
- nonstick cooking spray

for the filling:

- 6 large eggs
- 1 c. 36 percent heavy cream
- ½ c. mild cheddar cheese

STEP 1

Set the oven to 350 degrees F to preheat. Lightly coat a 9-inch pie pan with nonstick cooking spray and set it aside.

STEP 2

Prepare the crust a day ahead by combining all the ingredients in a bowl until the mixture turns into a dough. Transfer the dough onto the prepared pie pan and spread out until completely covered. If needed, transfer to the freezer and chill for 10 minutes to set.

STEP 3

Bake the crust for 25 minutes in the preheated oven until golden brown. Then, transfer to a cooling rack and let cool completely. Cover and refrigerate until ready to cook the quiche.

STEP 4

Prepare the quiche filling by combining the eggs, cheese, and heavy cream in a large bowl. Add a pinch of salt and mix well until smooth.

STEP 5

Pour the mixture into the prepared pie crust—Bake for 25 minutes, or until the quiche is just set. Insert a toothpick in the center of the quiche; if it comes out clean, it is ready.

STEP 6

Place the quiche on a cooling rack and allow it to sit for about 10 minutes. Slice and serve. Store in the refrigerator in an airtight container for up to 3 days.

NUTRITIONAL INFORMATION

166 Calories, 17g Fats, 2g Net Carbs, and 17g Protein

KETO GREEN EGGS

Cooking Difficulty: 2/10	Cooking Time: 9 minutes	Servings: 2

INGREDIENTS

- ¼ tsp. ground cayenne
- ¼ tsp. ground cumin
- 4 eggs
- ½ c. chopped parsley
- ½ c. chopped cilantro
- 1 tsp. thyme leaves
- 2 garlic cloves
- 1 tbsp. coconut oil
- 2 tbsps. butter

STEP 1

Melt the butter and coconut oil in a skillet before adding the garlic and frying.

STEP 2

Add in the thyme, parsley, and cilantro and cook another 3 minutes.

STEP 3

At this time, add in the eggs and season. Cover with a lid and let this cook for another 5 minutes before serving.

NUTRITIONAL INFORMATION

311 Calories, 27g Fats, 4g Net Carbs, 12.8 Protein

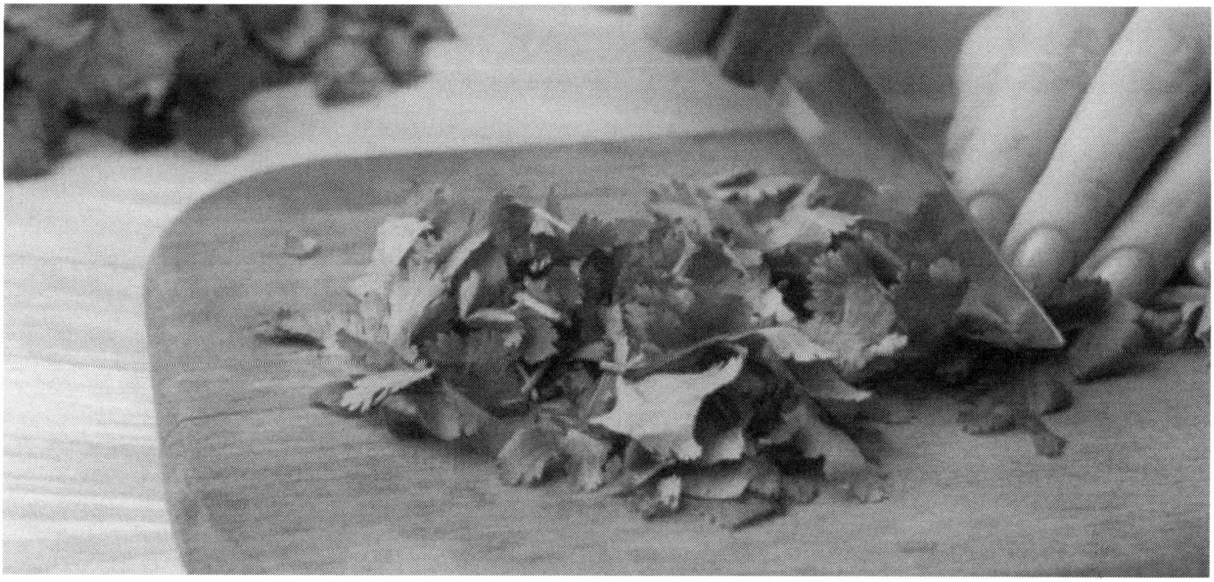

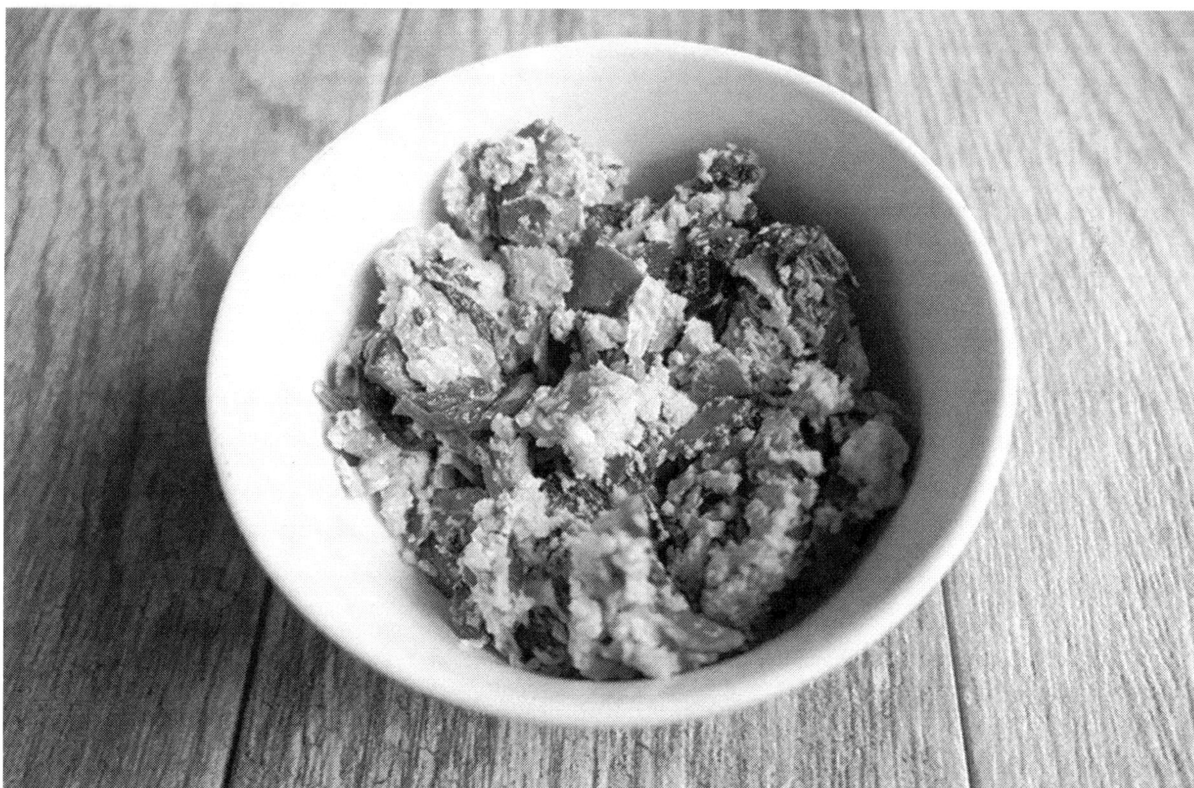

BACON AND RICOTTA BREAKFAST MUFFINS

Cooking Difficulty: 3/10	Cooking Time: 60 minutes	Servings: 6

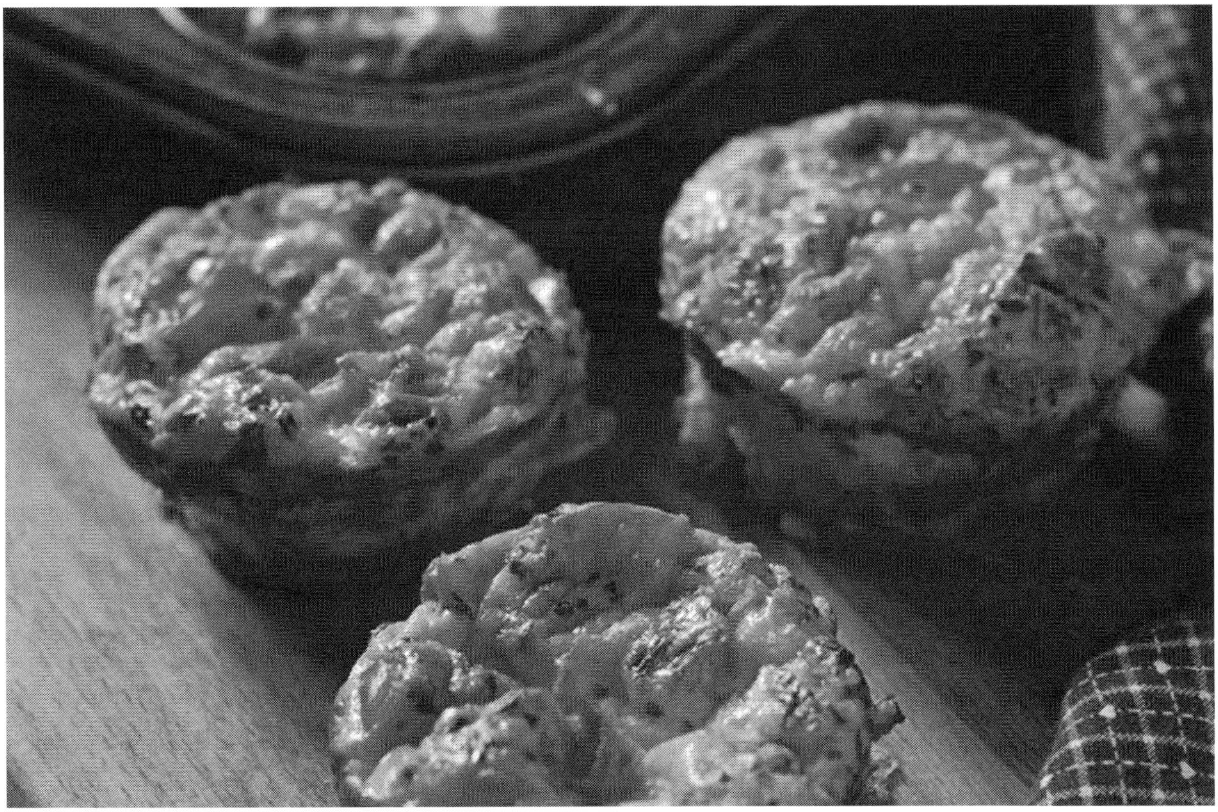

NUTRITIONAL INFORMATION

440 Calories, 29g Fats, 22g Net Carbs, 27g Protein

INGREDIENTS

- 2 large eggs
- 1 lb. ricotta cheese
- 10 oz. baby spinach, rinsed and drained thoroughly
- 7 oz. bacon
- 2 oz. chopped toasted pine nuts
- 1 c. freshly grated parmesan cheese
- ½ c. thick plain greek yogurt
- sea salt
- black pepper
- nonstick cooking spray

STEP 1

Set the oven to 350 degrees F to preheat. Lightly coat a 12 cup muffin tin with nonstick cooking spray and set it aside.

STEP 2

Bring a saucepan of water to a boil, then add the spinach and blanch for 30 minutcs or until wilted. Drain well and set aside in a colander.

STEP 3

Meanwhile, dice the bacon and set it aside.

STEP 4

Once the spinach is drained, finely chop, then transfer to a large bowl. Add the ricotta cheese, pine nuts, Parmesan cheese, yogurt, eggs, and bacon. Mix very well until evenly combined.

STEP 5

Divide the mixture among the muffin cups, then bake for 30 minutes or until golden brown.

STEP 6

Place on a cooling rack and allow to cool slightly. Store in an airtight container and refrigerate for up to 3 days, or freeze for up to 3 weeks. Reheat in the microwave before serving.

VANILLA SMOOTHIE

Cooking Difficulty: 1/10	Cooking Time: 3 minutes	Servings: 1

INGREDIENTS

- whipped cream
- 3 drops liquid stevia
- ¼ tsp. vanilla
- 4 ice cubes
- ¼ c. water
- ½ c. mascarpone cheese
- 2 egg yolks

STEP 1

Take out your blender and add in all the ingredients.

STEP 2

Place the lid on top and blend. When the ingredients are well mixed, pour into a glass and serve.

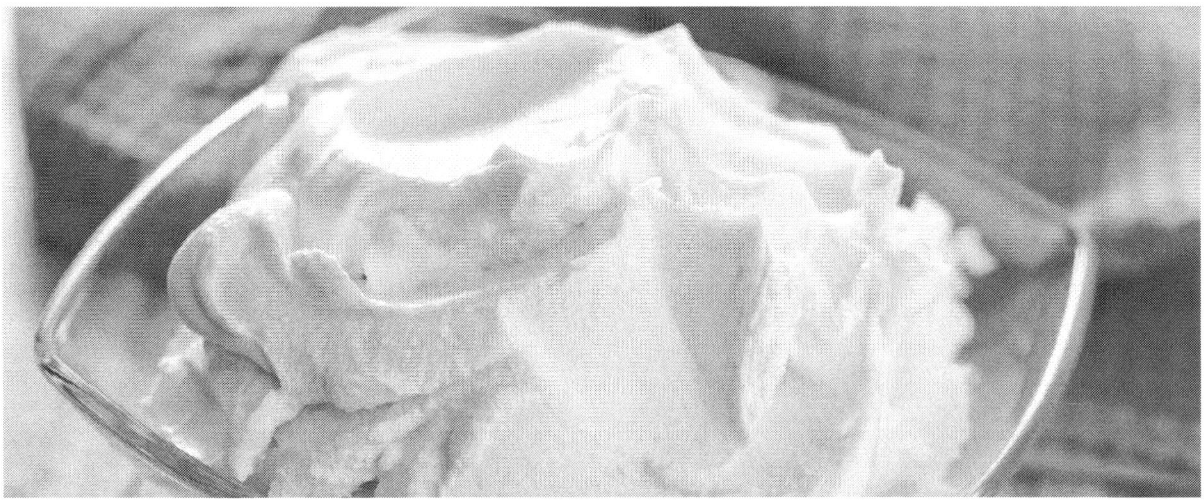

NUTRITIONAL INFORMATION

650 Calories, 64g Fats, 4g Net Carbs, and 12g Protein

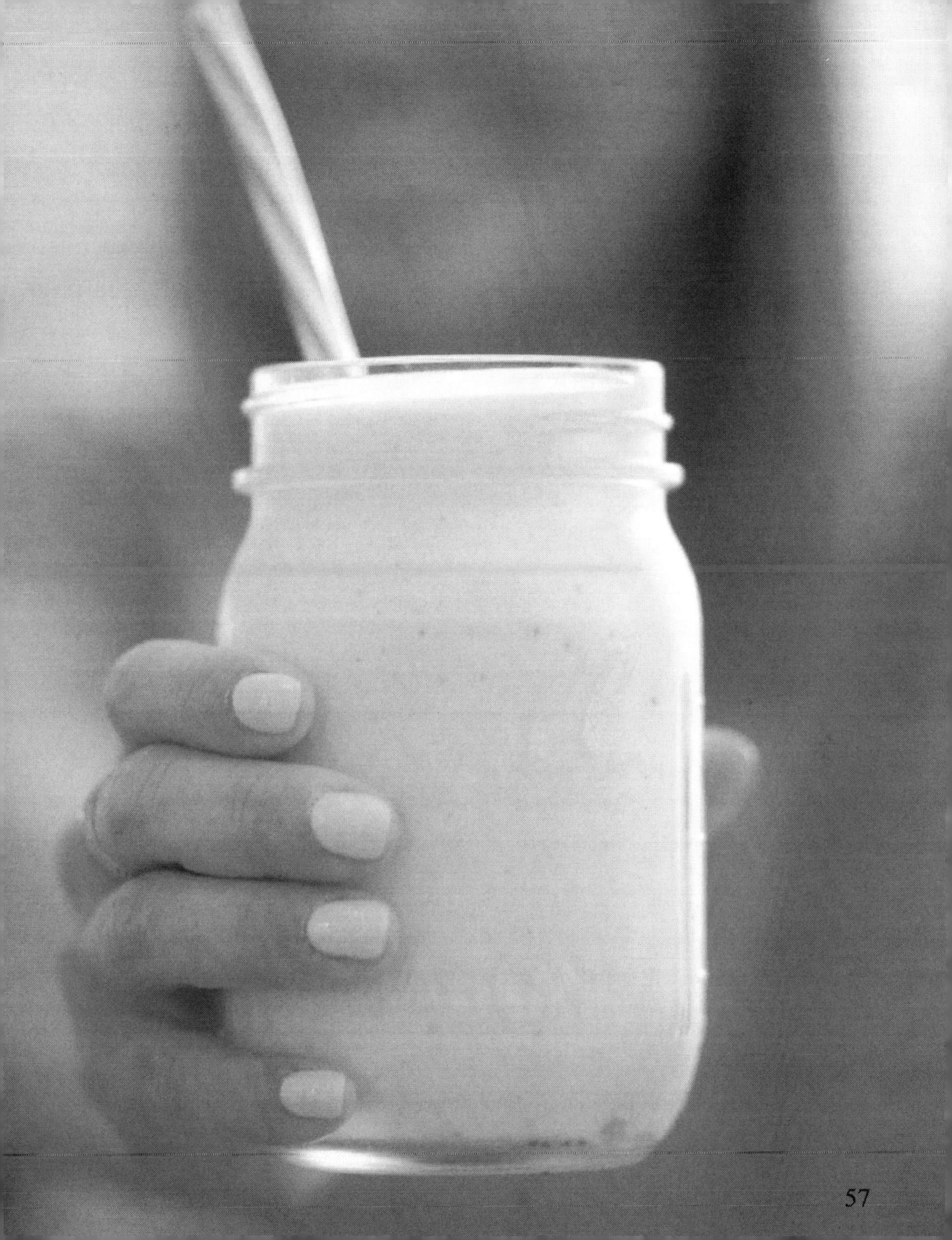

COCONUT PANCAKES

Cooking Difficulty: 2/10	Cooking Time: 22 minutes	Servings: 2

INGREDIENTS

- 4 tbsps. maple syrup
- ¼ c. shredded coconut
- salt
- ½ tbsp. erythritol
- 1 tsp. cinnamon
- 1tbsp. almond flour
- 2 oz. cream cheese
- 2 eggs

STEP 1

Beat the eggs together before adding in the almond flour and cream cheese.

STEP 2

Now add in the rest of the ingredients and stir until well combined.

STEP 3

Take out a frying pan and fry the pancakes on both sides. Add to a plate and sprinkle some coconut on top.

NUTRITIONAL INFORMATION

575 Calories, 51g Fats, 3.5g Net Carbs, 19g Protein

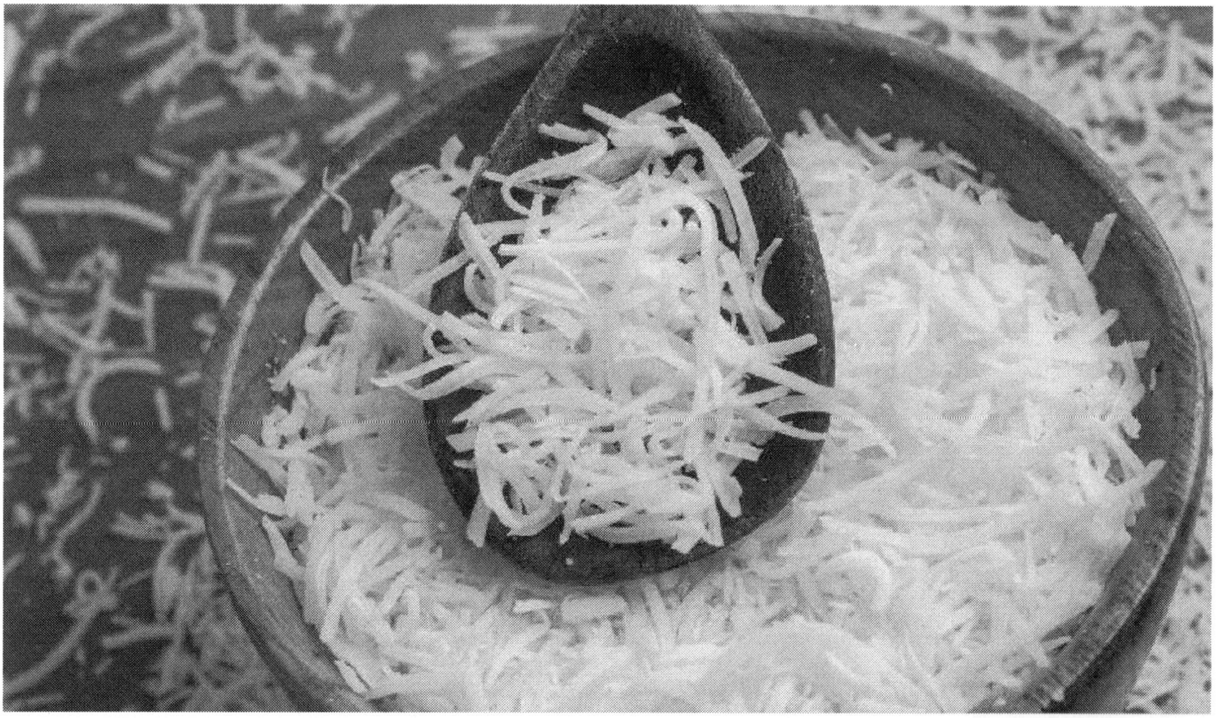

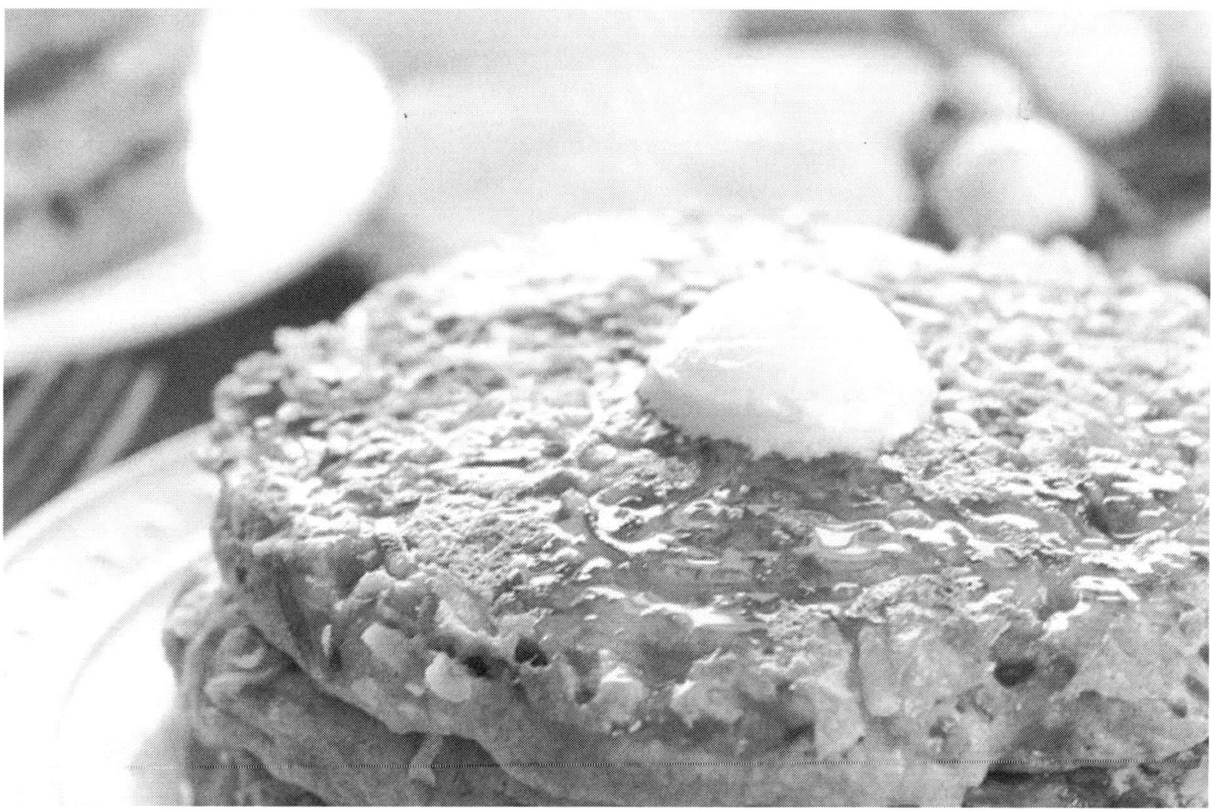

CHOCOLATE AND PEANUT BUTTER MUFFINS

Cooking Difficulty: 2/10	Cooking Time: 27 minutes	Servings: 6

INGREDIENTS

- 2 eggs
- 1/3 c. almond milk
- 1/3 c. peanut butter
- salt
- 1 tsp. baking powder
- ½ c. erythritol
- 1 c. almond flour
- 80g cacao nibs

STEP 1

Bring out a bowl and mix the salt, baking powder, erythritol, and almond flour together. Add the eggs, almond milk, and peanut butter next.

STEP 2

Finally, mix in the cacao nibs before pouring this into a muffin tin.

STEP 3

Allow the oven to heat up to 350 degrees F. Place the muffin tray into the oven to bake.

STEP 4

After 25 minutes, the muffins are done, and you can store them.

NUTRITIONAL INFORMATION

265 Calories, 20.5g Fats, 2g Net Carbs, 7.5g Protein

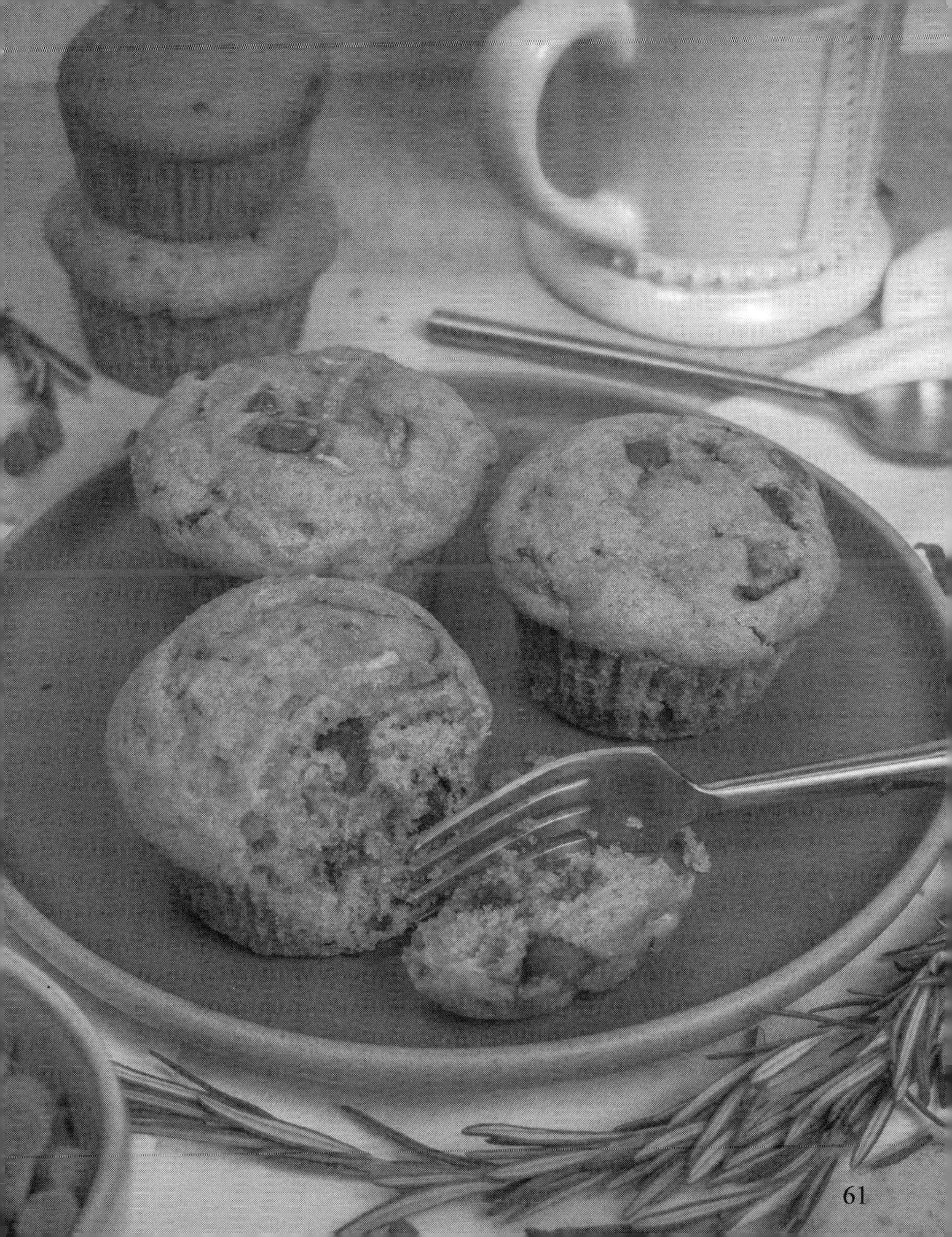

CREAMY HERBED-BAKED EGGS

Cooking Difficulty: 3/10	Cooking Time: 27 minutes	Servings: 4

INGREDIENTS

- 4 large eggs
- 60 grams 36 percent heavy cream
- 2 tbsps. grass-fed butter, at room temperature
- 4 tsps. chopped fresh parsley
- 4 tsps. chopped fresh chives
- sea salt
- black pepper

STEP 1

Set the oven to 350 degrees F to preheat. Use 1 tablespoon of butter to coat four 1-cup ovenproof ramekins.

STEP 2

Crack an egg into each ramekin, then divide the heavy cream among them. Top with the fresh parsley and chives. Season with salt and pepper.

STEP 3

Arrange the ramekins on a baking sheet and bake for 20 minutes, or until the eggs are set.

STEP 4

Transfer to a cooling rack and let stand for 5 minutes before serving. To store, cover with aluminum foil and refrigerate for up to 2 days. Reheat in the microwave before serving.

NUTRITIONAL INFORMATION

158 Calories, 16g Fats, 1g Net Carbs, 3g Protein

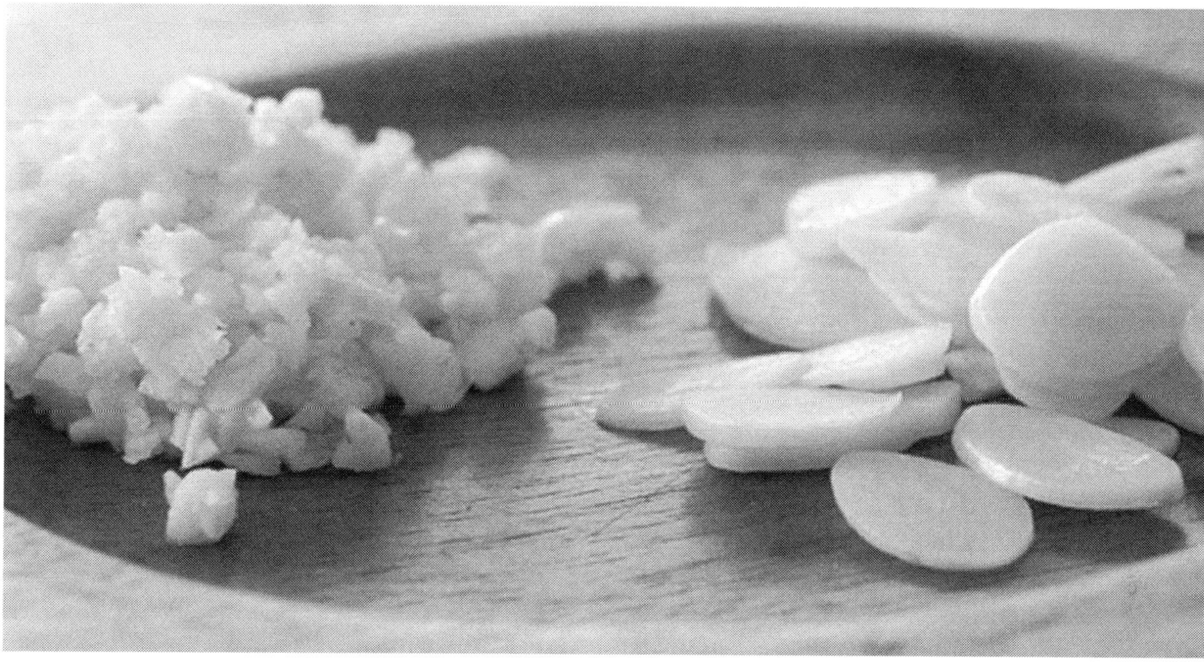

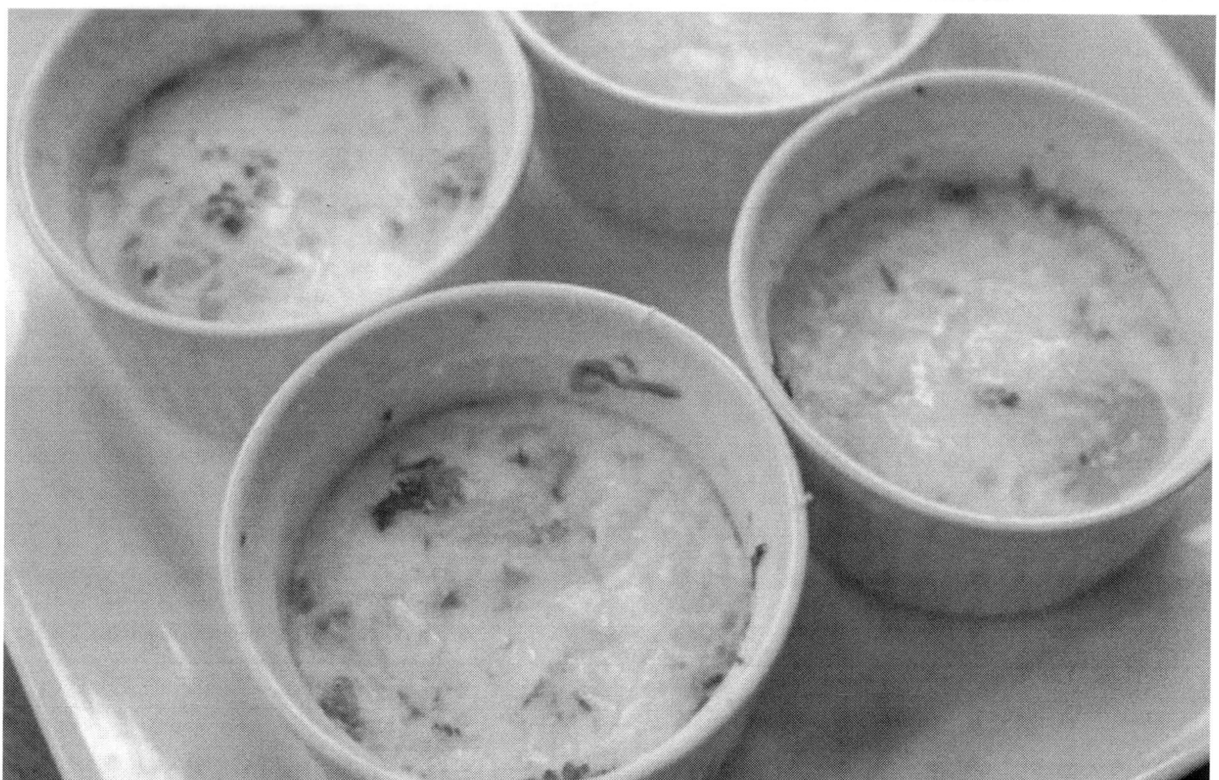

LUNCH RECIPES

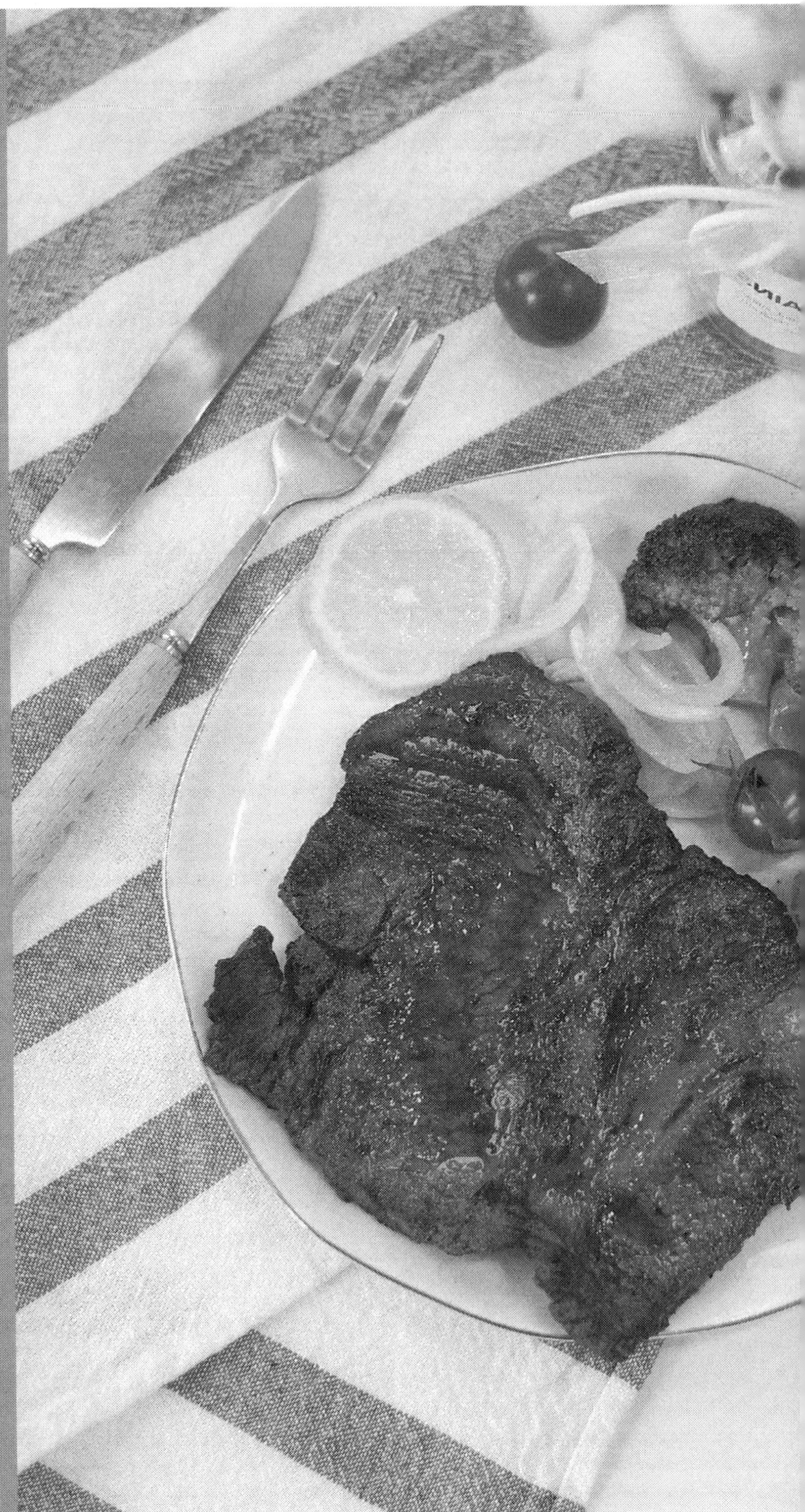

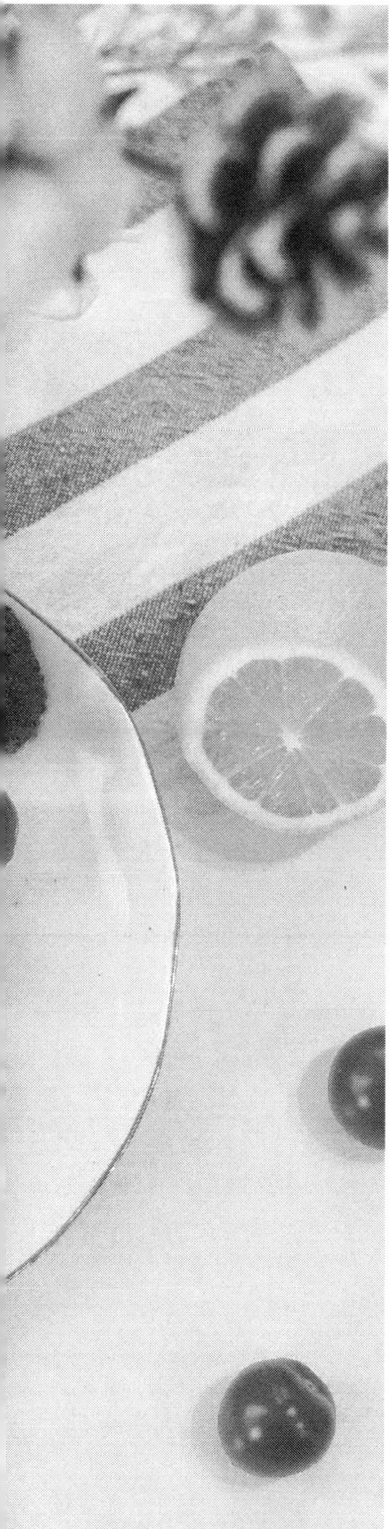

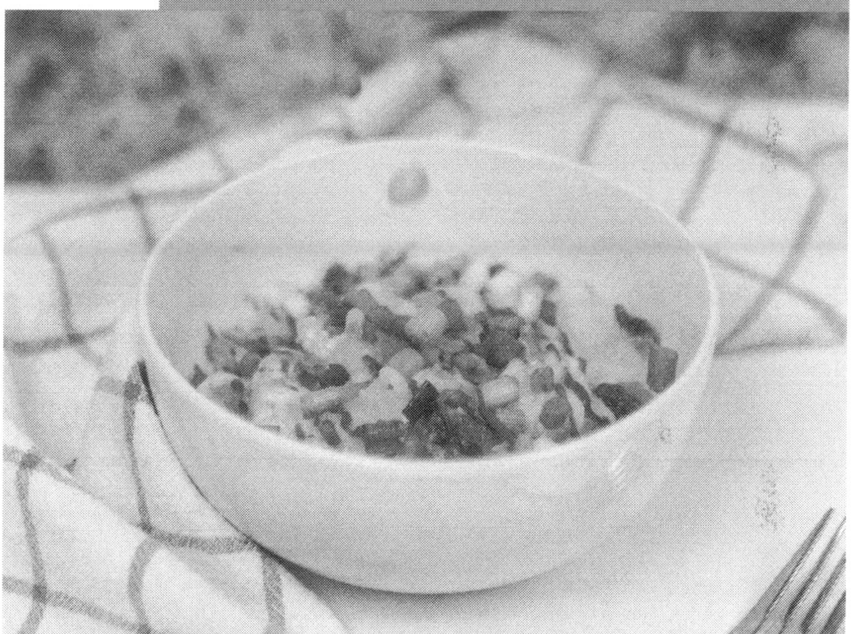

CHILI ORANGE SHRIMP

Cooking Difficulty: 1/10	Cooking Time: 6 minutes	Servings: 4

INGREDIENTS

- 2 lb peeled and deveined shrimp
- 2/3 c. cream
- 1 chipotle chili
- 1 tsp. orange zest
- cinnamon
- 5 spice
- salt
- pepper

STEP 1

Blend the half and half, chili, orange, salt, and pepper.

STEP 2

Put in a frying pan with the shrimp. Sautee 5 minutes

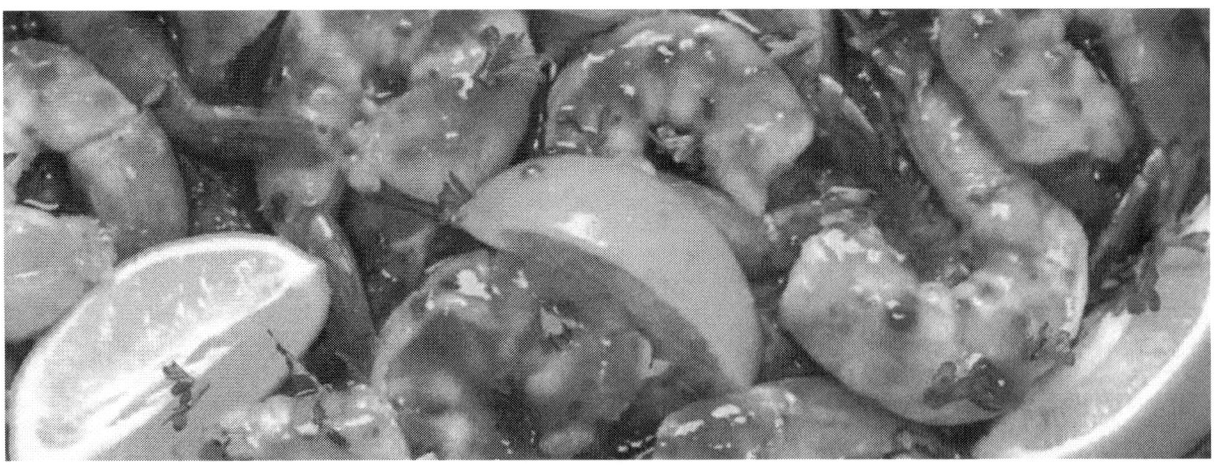

NUTRITIONAL INFORMATION

186 Calories, 6g Fats, 3g Net Carbs, and 28g Protein.

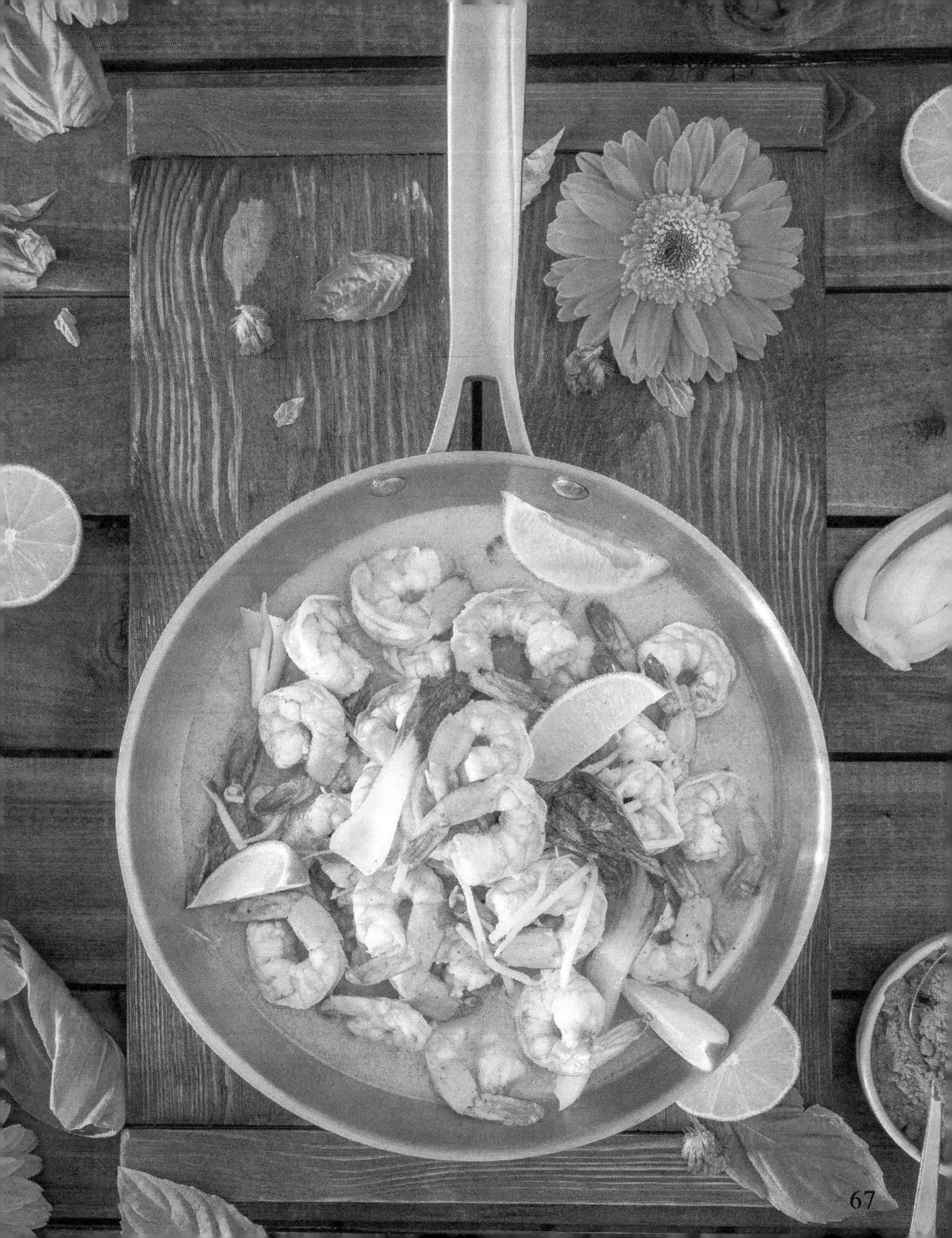

STICKY DRUMSTICKS

Cooking Difficulty: 3/10	Cooking Time: 55 minutes	Servings: 4

INGREDIENTS

- chicken drumsticks
- ½ c. olive oil
- ¼ c. sweet chili sauce
- 2 garlic cloves, minced
- ¼ c. soy sauce
- 2 tsps. sesame seeds

STEP 1

Slice through the thickest part of each drumstick using a sharp knife. Arrange them in a glass dish.

STEP 2

In a bowl, mix the sauces and garlic. Rub all over the drumstick; marinate for about 30 minutes in the refrigerator.

STEP 3

Preheat the oven to 248 degrees F of 356 for the fan.

STEP 4

Place the drumsticks on a nonstick baking paper. Sprinkle them with sesame seeds. Bake for about 45 minutes. Let cool slightly; serve.

NUTRITIONAL INFORMATION

144 Calories, 10g Fats, 2g Net Carbs, 8.5g Protein

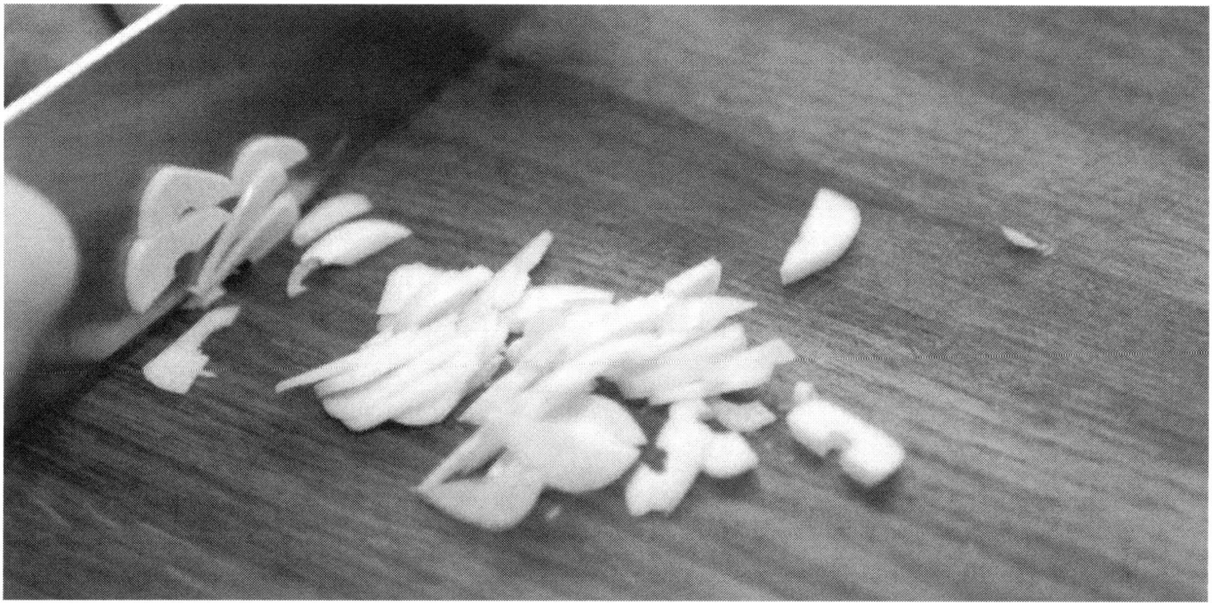

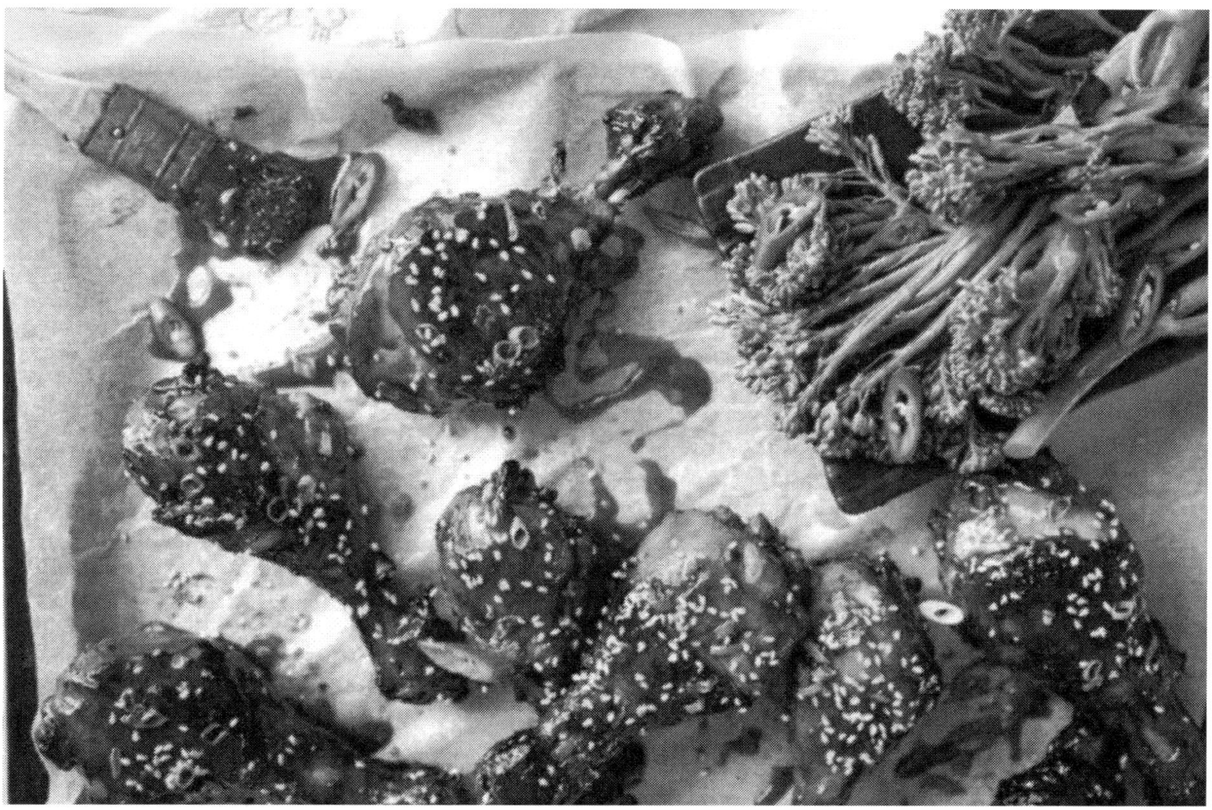

HAM, ONION AND GREEN BEAN SALAD

Cooking Difficulty: 2/10	Cooking Time: 5 minutes	Servings: 3

INGREDIENTS

- ½ lb. trimmed green beans
- 1 minced white onion
- 1 diced roasted red bell pepper
- 1 oz. chopped spanish ham
- 1 chopped hardboiled egg
- 2½ tbsps. fresh flat-leaf parsley
- 2 tbsps. extra virgin olive oil
- 1½ tbsps. red wine vinegar
- sea salt
- black pepper

STEP 1

Rinse and drain the steamed green beans. Blot dry with paper towels and set aside.

STEP 2

Combine the olive oil, vinegar, and a dash of salt and pepper. Mix well.

STEP 3

Divide the green beans into individual servings, followed by the minced onion, ham, peppers, egg, and parsley. Add the dressing.

STEP 4

Cover and refrigerate for up to 2 days. Reheat before serving, if desired.

NUTRITIONAL INFORMATION

144 Calories, 10g Fats, 2g Net Carbs, 8.5g Protein

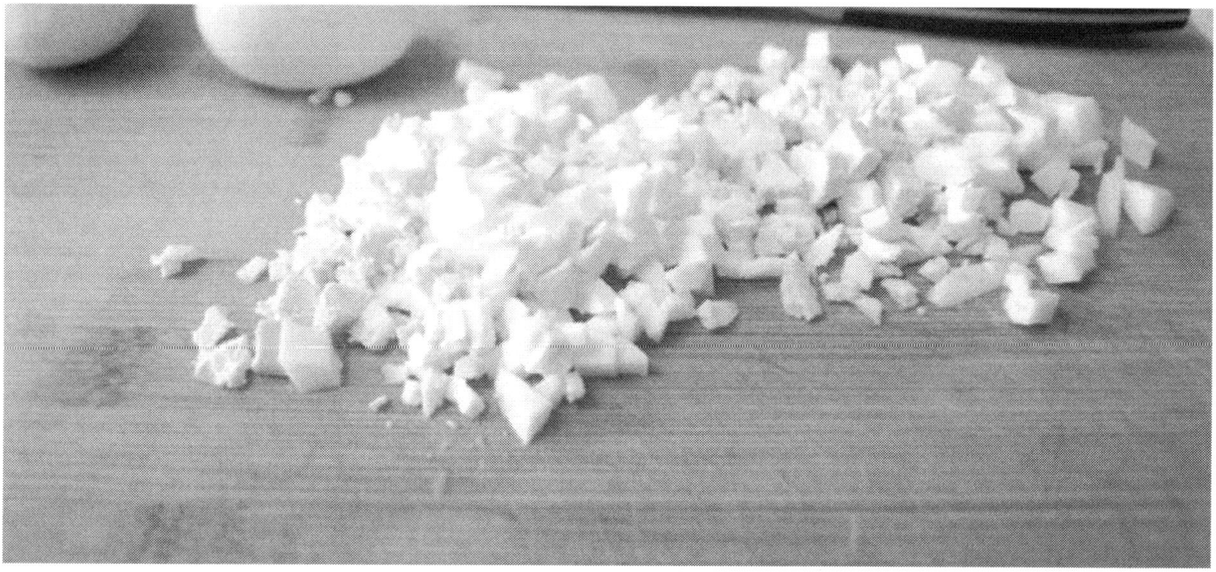

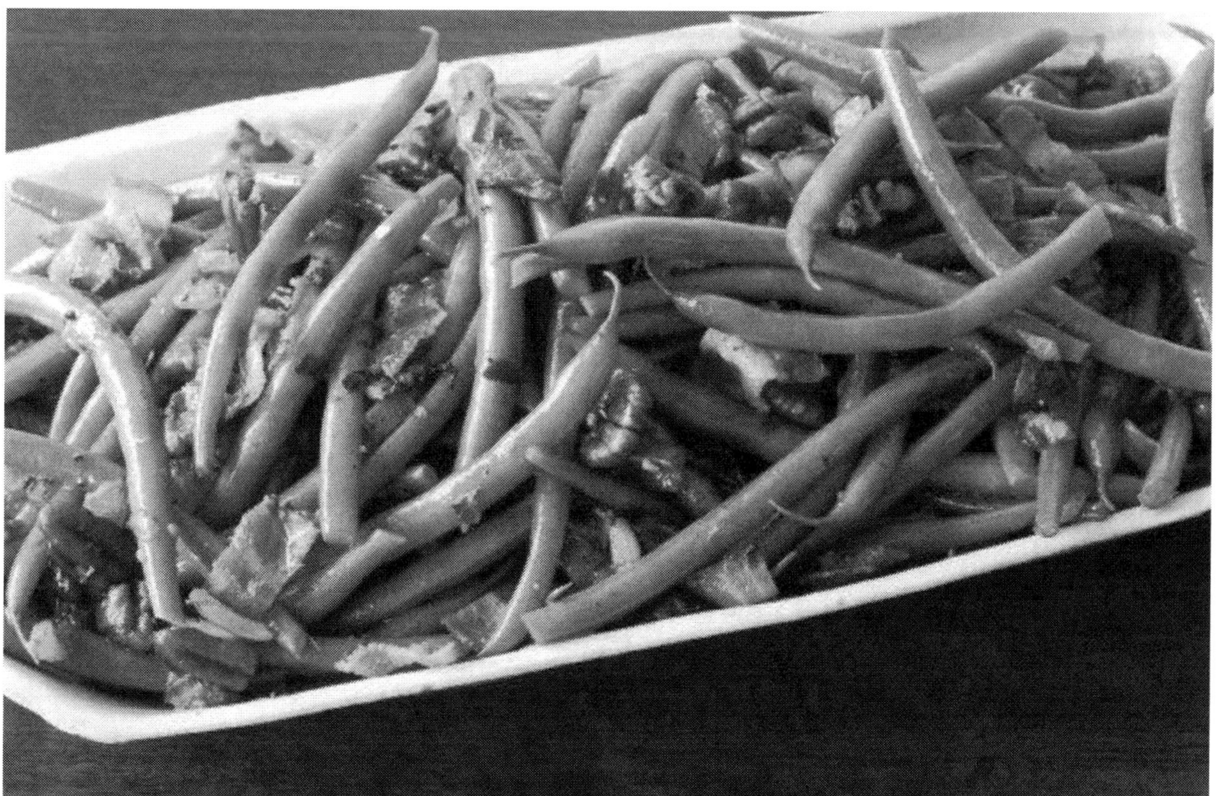

LAMB SPINACH ROGAN JOSH

Cooking Difficulty: 2/10	Cooking Time: 240 minutes	Servings: 6

INGREDIENTS

- 2½ lb. diced lamb
- 2 sliced red onions
- 1 c. greek yogurt
- 2 tbsps. ghee
- rogan josh curry paste
- salt
- pepper

STEP 1

Mix all ingredients together in a pot.

STEP 2

Add a little water and simmer for 4 hours.

STEP 3

Serve.

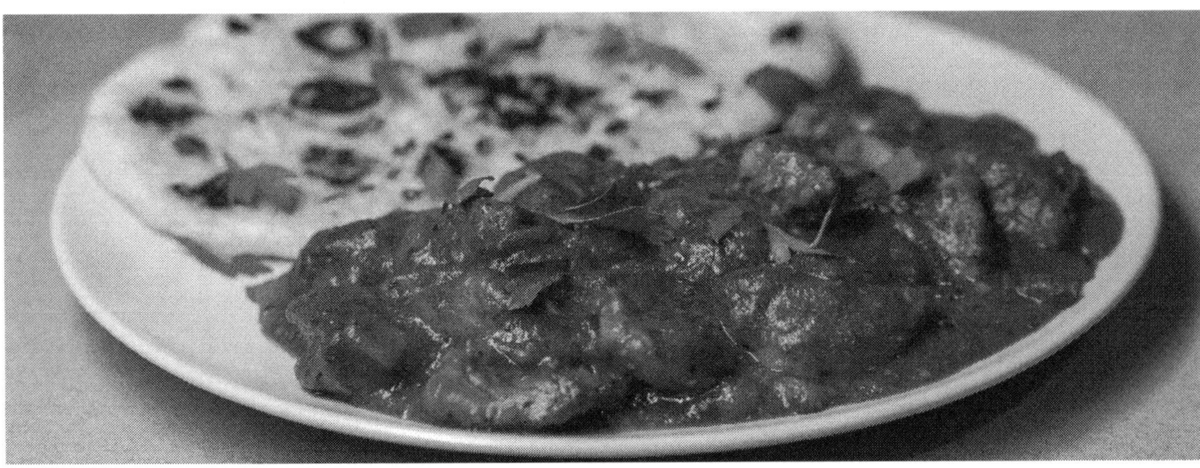

NUTRITIONAL INFORMATION

450 Calories, 28g Fats, 4g Net Carbs, 38g Protein

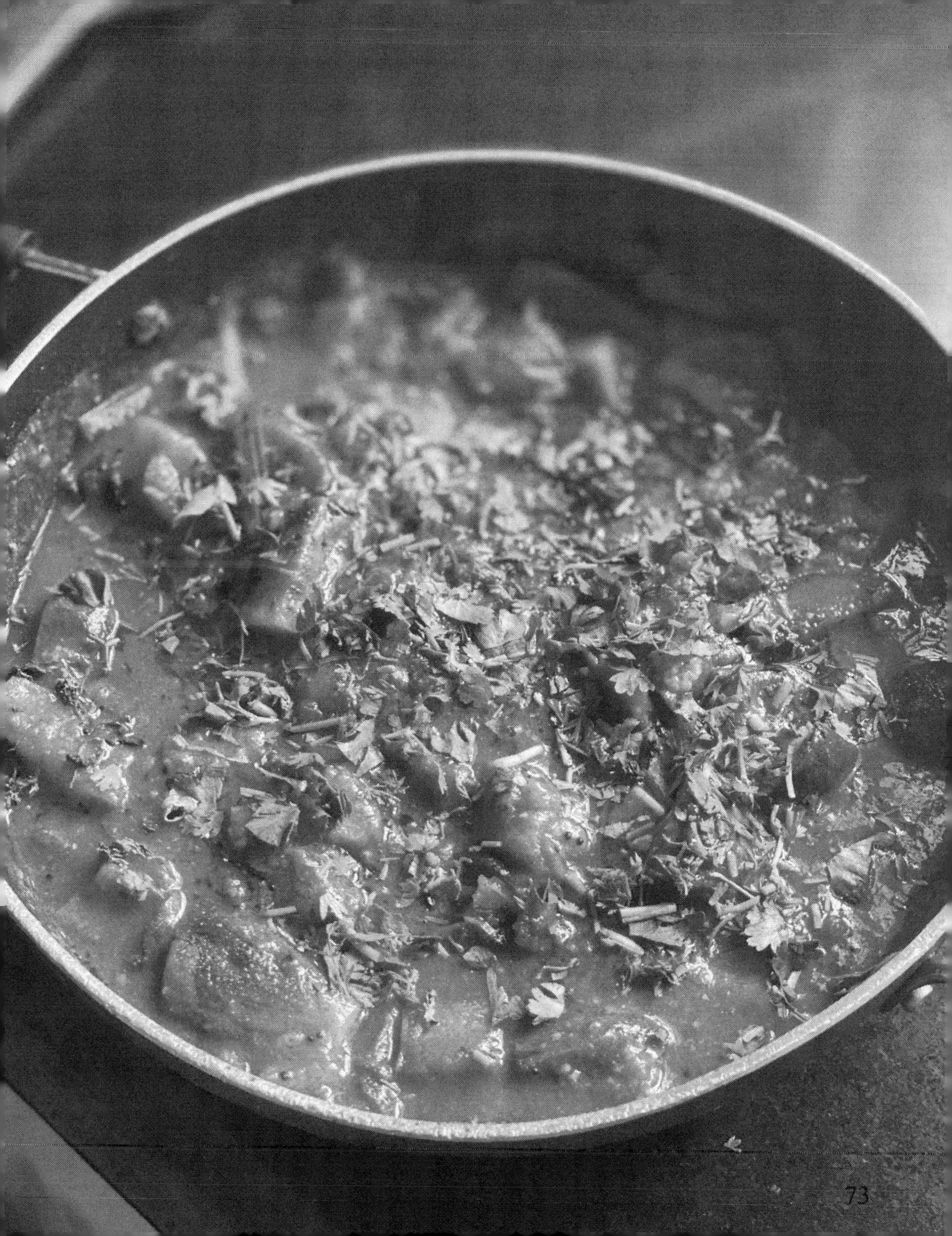

SPICY GARLIC BUTTER SHRIMP

Cooking Difficulty: 4/10	Cooking Time: 35 minutes	Servings: 5

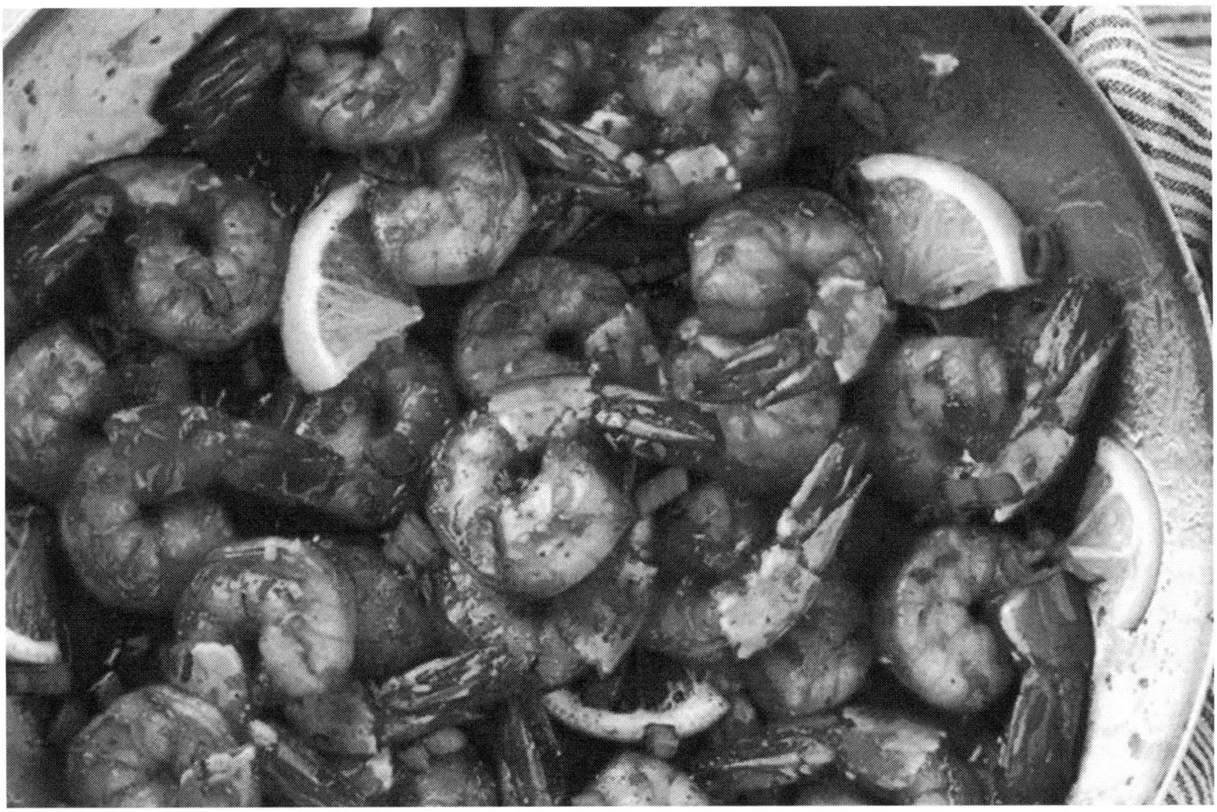

NUTRITIONAL INFORMATION

300 Calories, 11g Fats, 5g Net Carbs, 10g Protein

INGREDIENTS

- lbs. large-sized shrimp, unpeeled
- 2 tbsps. garlic, minced
- ½ c. butter
- lemon pepper seasoning
- garlic powder

STEP 1

Preheat the oven to 300 degrees F.

STEP 2

Mix the butter and the garlic.

STEP 3

Place the shrimp in a saucepan and dot with the garlic butter; sprinkle well with the garlic powder and the lemon pepper.

STEP 4

In an open state, bake for about 30 minutes, stirring once or twice, until the shrimp are opaque, making sure the shrimp is evenly cooked.

STEP 5

Serve alongside the butter sauce that is in a separate bowl or the one containing the shrimp for dipping.

STEP 6

You may serve alongside cauliflower rice.

BURGER WITH AVOCADO

Cooking Difficulty: 3/10	Cooking Time: 12 minutes	Servings: 2

INGREDIENTS

- ½ lb. 85 percent lean ground beef
- 1 small avocado
- 2 slices yellow cheddar cheese
- sea salt
- black pepper

STEP 1

Preheat the broiler or grill to high.

STEP 2

Divide the ground beef into two equal-sized patties—season with salt and pepper.

STEP 3

Grill or broil the beef patties for about 5 minutes per side or until cooked through.

STEP 4

Transfer the patties to a platter and add the cheese. To store, wrap in aluminum foil and refrigerate for up to 3 days.

STEP 5

Right before serving, reheat the burger patty in a microwave oven. Slice the avocado into thin strips and place on top of the patty. Serve warm.

NUTRITIONAL INFORMATION

502 Calories, 38.2 g Fat, 1.1 g Carbs, 38.1 g Protein

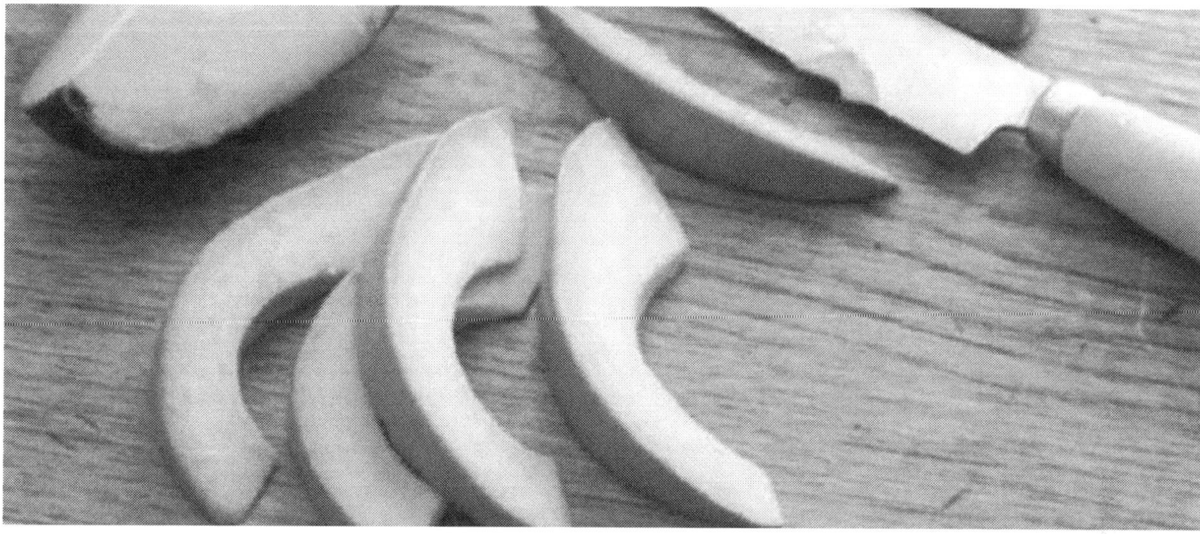

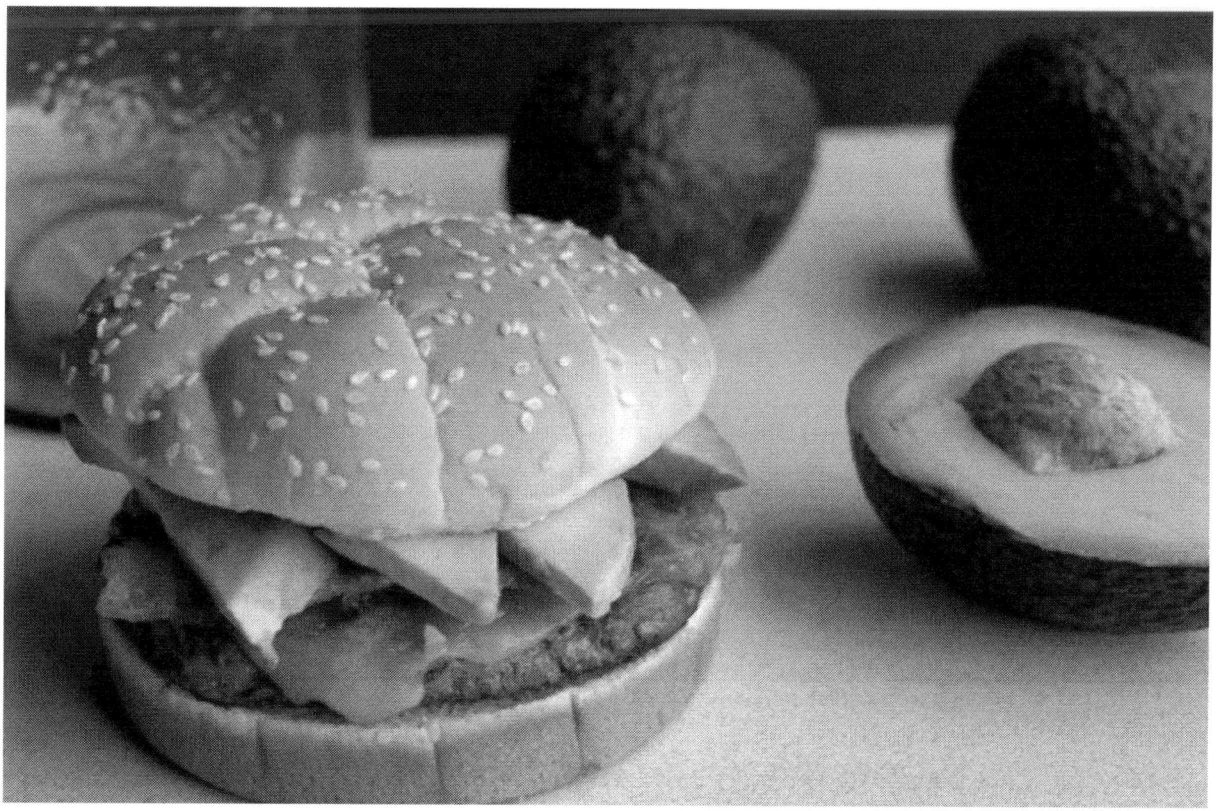

MUSHROOM AND SPAGHETTI SQUASH CASSEROLE

Cooking Difficulty: 5/10	Cooking Time: 97 minutes	Servings: 10

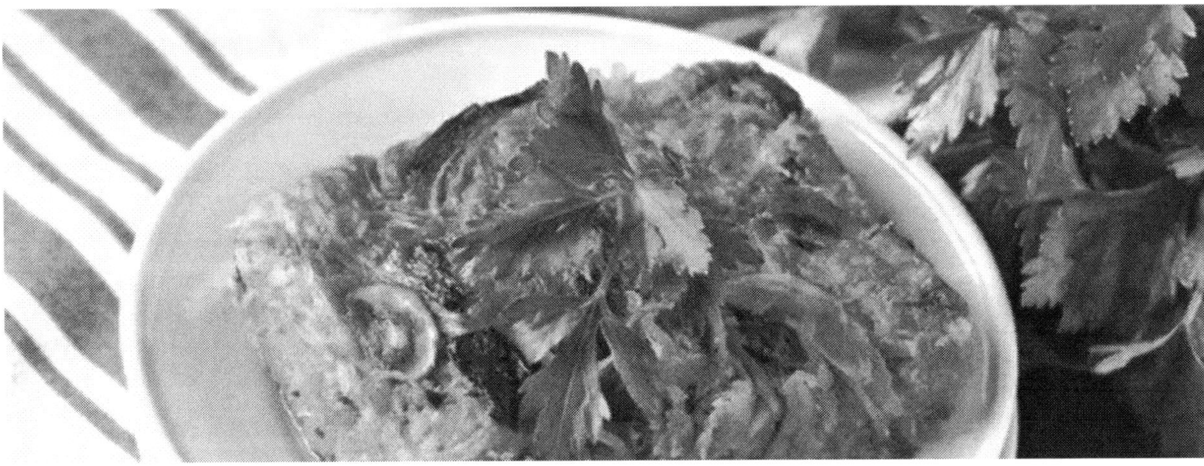

INGREDIENTS

- 1 large spaghetti squash
- 1 minced onion
- ½ lb. lean organic ground beef
- ½ lb. italian sausage
- ½ lb. chicken or turkey sausage
- ½ lb. sliced mushrooms
- 18 oz. diced tomatoes
- 8 oz. grated parmesan cheese
- 6 oz. organic tomato paste
- 4 oz. mozzarella cheese
- 4 oz. ricotta cheese
- ½ c. butter
- ½ c. red wine
- ½ tsp. sea salt
- ½ tsp. black pepper

NUTRITIONAL INFORMATION

402 Calories, 24g Fats, 15g Net Carbs, 31g Protein

STEP 1
Set the oven to 350 degrees F to preheat.

STEP 2
Pierce, the spaghetti squash all over with a sharp, then place in the microwave and microwave on high for about 20 minutes. Set aside to cool.

STEP 3
Melt the butter in a skillet over medium-high flame. Sauté the ground beef and sausages until cooked through and crumbled.

STEP 4
Add the red wine and simmer until the liquid is reduced. Then, stir in the onion and garlic. Sauté until tender.

STEP 5
Add the mushrooms and sauté until tender. Stir in the diced tomatoes, tomato paste, and seasonings. Sauté until combined.

STEP 6
Halve the spaghetti squash and scrape out the flesh. Set aside.

STEP 7
Spread half the spaghetti squash in a baking dish, then add 2 ounces each of the mozzarella and ricotta, followed by 4 ounces of the Parmesan.

STEP 8
Spoon some tomato sauce on top, then add the remaining spaghetti squash. Add the remaining cheeses, then cover the dish.

STEP 9
Bake for 20 minutes, then uncover and bake for an additional 20 minutes.

STEP 10
Set the oven to broil and broil the casserole for 3 minutes, or until the top is browned and crisp.

STEP 11
Place on a cooling rack and let sit for 15 minutes. Slice into 10 equal servings, then cover and refrigerate for up to 5 days. Reheat before serving.

KETO CUBANO

Cooking Difficulty: 2/10	Cooking Time: 10 minutes	Servings: 4

INGREDIENTS

- bib lettuce
- 2 tbsps. dijon mustard
- 2 tbsps. mayo
- 1 tbsp. melted butter
- ¼ lb. sliced swiss cheese
- 1/3 lb. cooked pork tenderloin
- 1/3 lb. sliced cooked ham
- sliced dill pickles

STEP 1

Mix together the mustard and the mayo and spread over the lettuce.

STEP 2

Divide up the meats, cheese, and pickle between the sandwiches and roll them up tightly.

STEP 3

Serve right away.

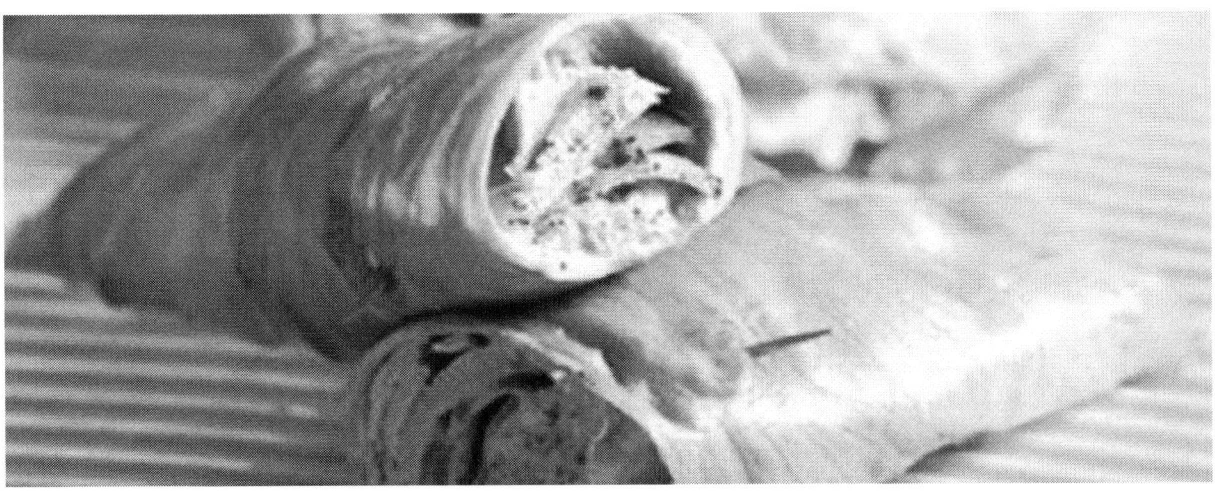

NUTRITIONAL INFORMATION

472 Calories, 36g Fats, 7g Net Carbs, and 28g Protein.

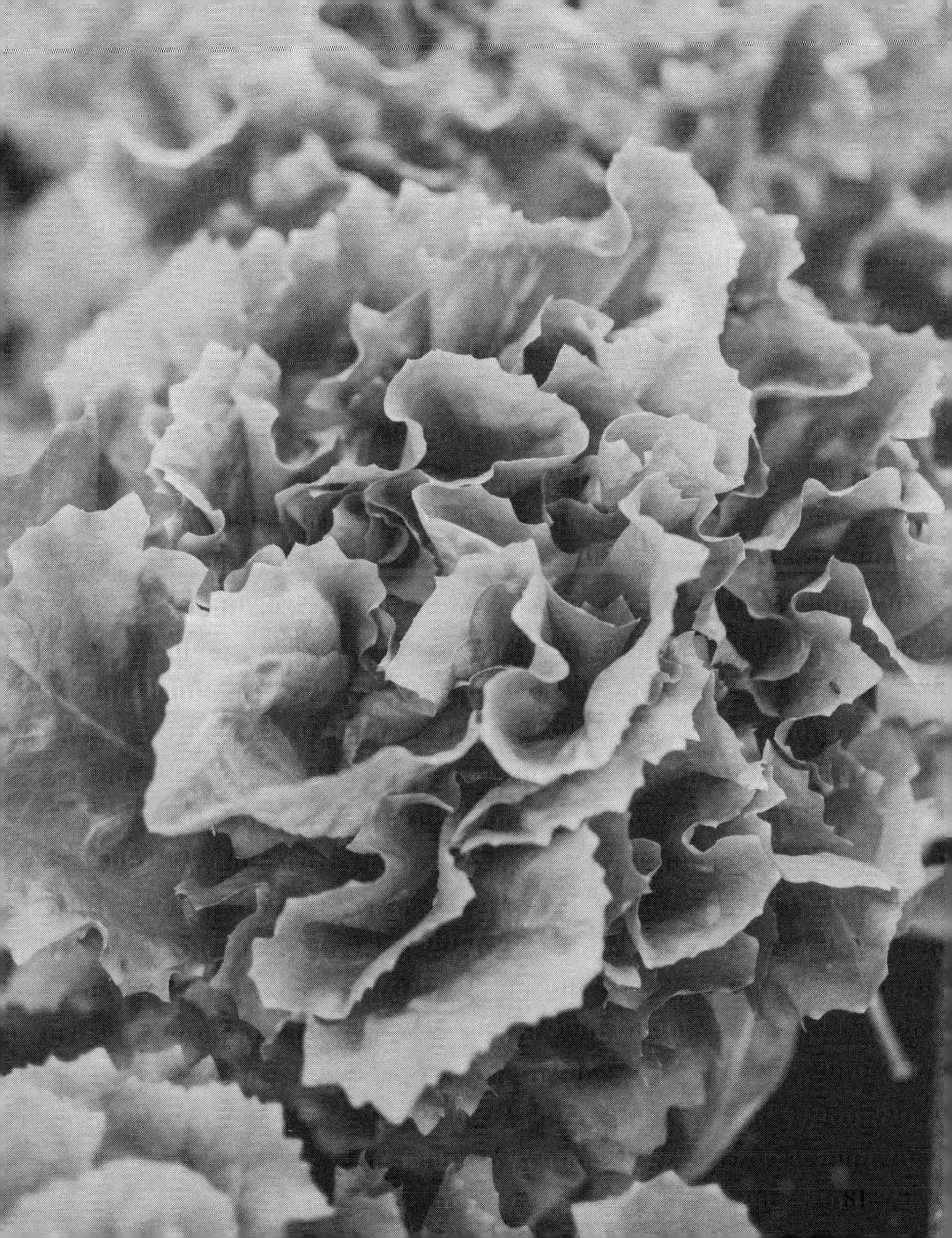

FETA CHEESE SALAD

Cooking Difficulty: 3/10	Cooking Time: 27 minutes	Servings: 8

INGREDIENTS

- 2 chopped spring onions
- 50g roasted pistachios
- 150g feta cheese
- 1 diced red onion
- 8 beetroots
- 4 tsps. balsamic vinegar
- 2 tsps. chutney
- 3 tsps. mayo

STEP 1

Add the beetroot and water to a pan and let it boil, cooking the beetroot for 20 minutes. Wash with cold water and remove the skin before slicing.

STEP 2

Mix the beetroot and onion together.

STEP 3

Now work on the dressing. Add the balsamic vinegar, mayo, and chutney together.

STEP 4

Take out a platter and add the vegetables and pour the dressing on top. Garnish with the onion and pecans and serve over feta cheese.

NUTRITIONAL INFORMATION

413 Calories, 31.9g Fats, 28.2g Net Carbs,7.2gProtein

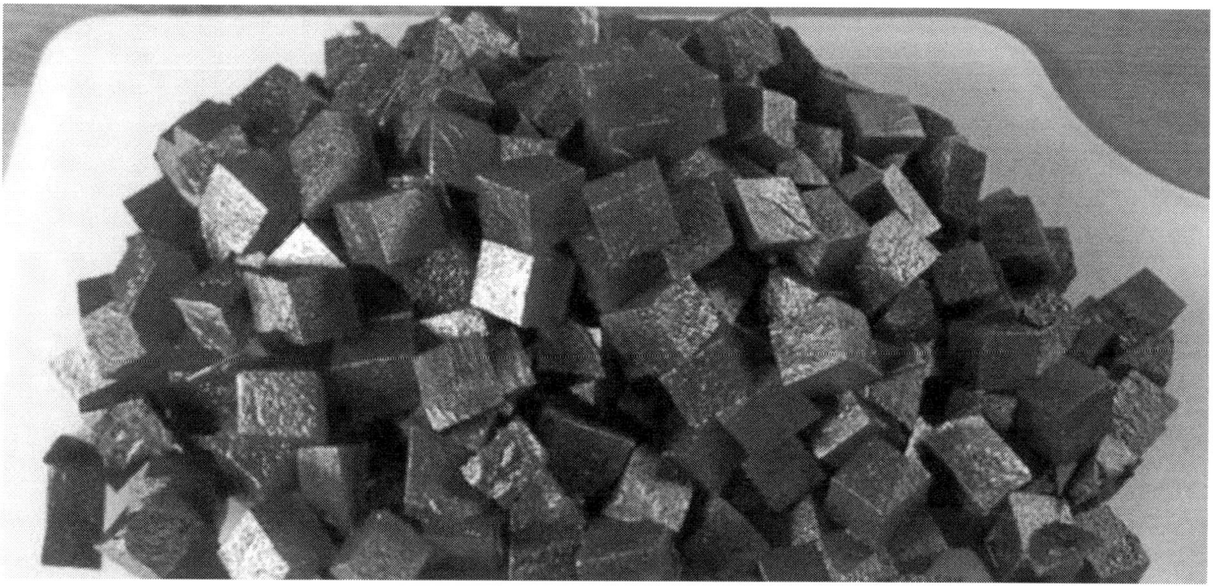

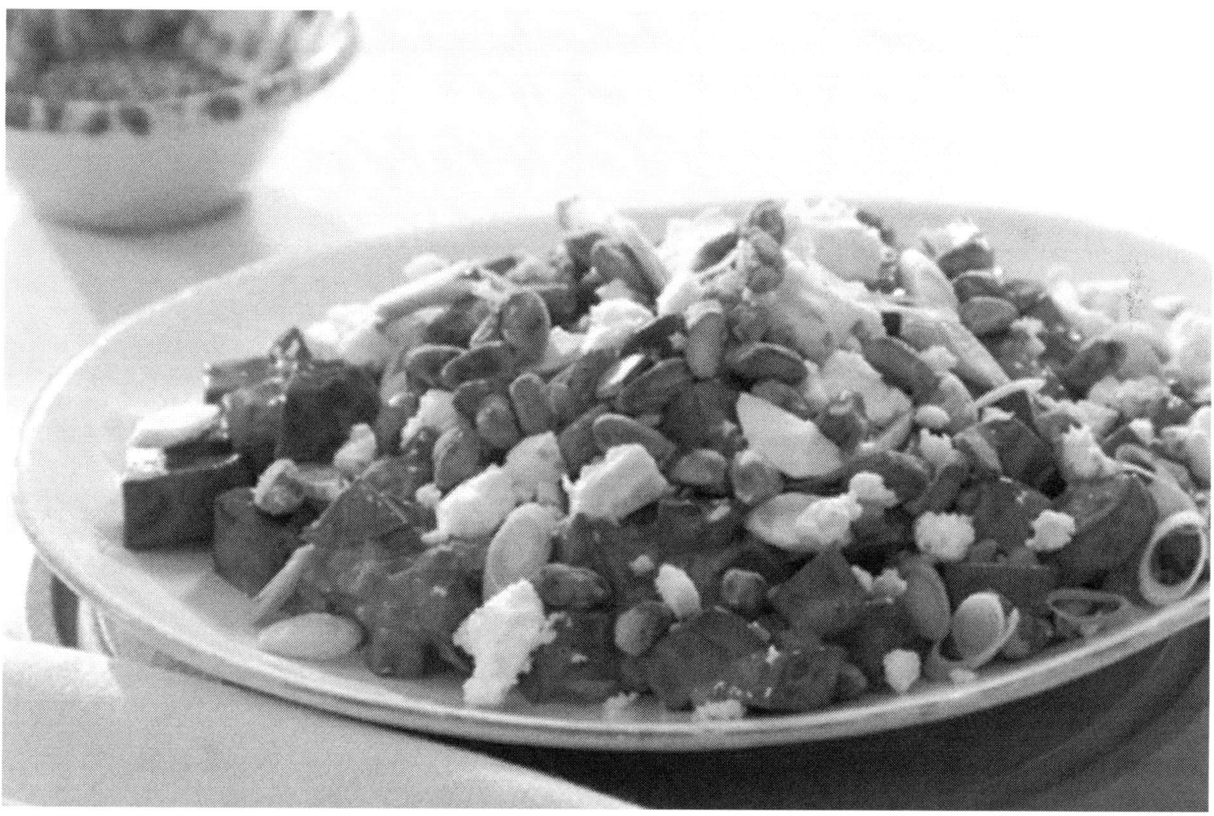

EASY GRILLED SHRIMP WITH AVOCADO AND TOMATO

Cooking Difficulty: 3/10	Cooking Time: 12 minutes	Servings: 6

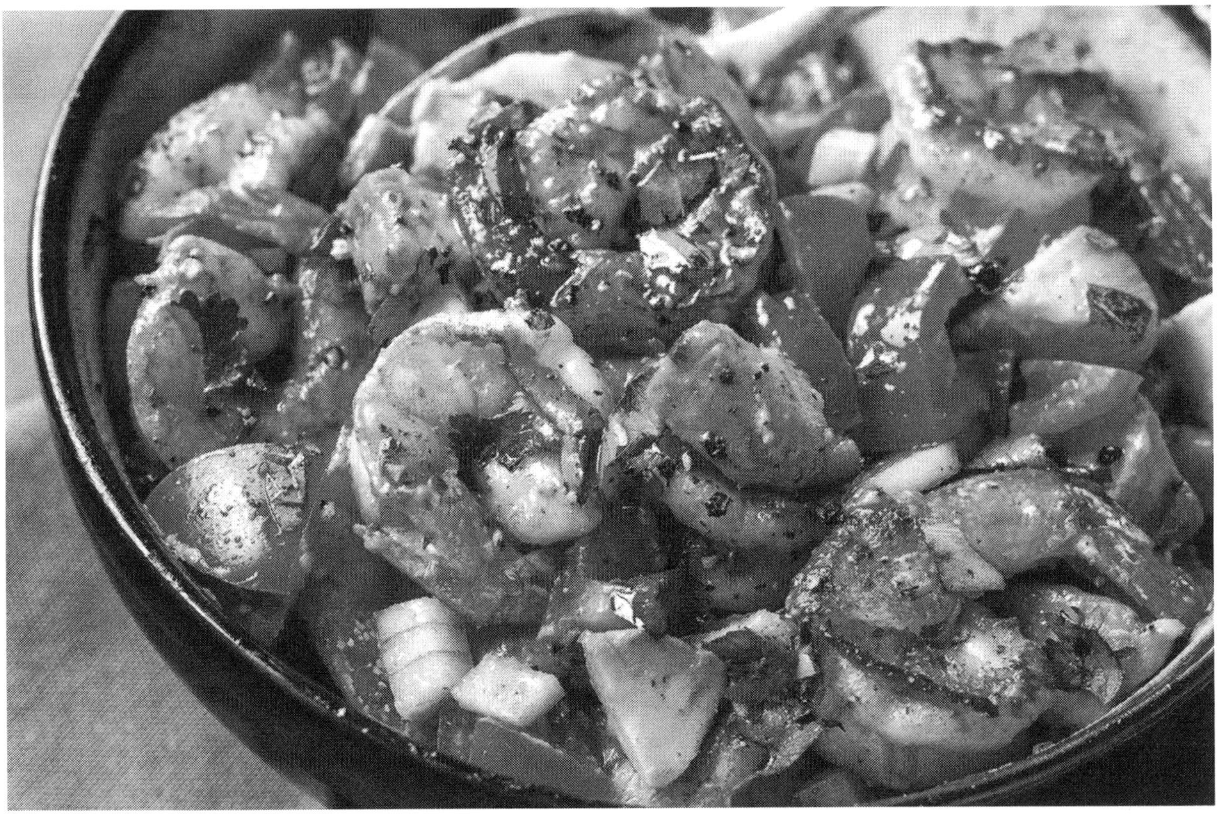

NUTRITIONAL INFORMATION

300 Calories, 11g Fats, 5g Net Carbs, 10g Protein

INGREDIENTS

- 2 cubed avocados
- 2 lb. deveined shrimp
- ½ c. chopped tomato
- ½ c. chopped bell pepper
- ½ c. chopped onion
- 4 tbsps. olive oil
- 2 tsps. squeezed lime juice
- 1 tsp. garlic powder
- 1 tsp. fine sea salt
- ¼ tsp. black pepper

STEP 1

Place a grill over medium-high flame and heat through.

STEP 2

Meanwhile, combine the garlic powder, half the salt and pepper, and olive oil in a large bowl. Add the shrimp and toss well to coat. Set aside.

STEP 3

In a salad bowl, combine the bell pepper, tomato, onion, avocado, and lime juice. Season with the remaining salt and toss gently to coat. Cover and refrigerate until ready to serve.

STEP 4

Cook the shrimp in the hot grill for 3 minutes per side, or until cooked through.

STEP 5

Divide the shrimp into individual servings, followed by the salad. Cover and refrigerate for up to 3 days. Reheat the shrimp before serving.

SAVORY BEEF BALLS WITH ASIAN STYLE DIP

STEP 1

Set the oven to 425 degrees F to preheat. Lightly coat a baking sheet with nonstick cooking spray and set aside.

STEP 2

Place the ground beef in a large mixing bowl and add the egg, onion, salt, garlic, and a generous pinch of black pepper. Mix everything well with clean hands.

STEP 3

Make about 40 1-inch sized balls from the meat mixture and arrange them on the prepared baking sheet.

STEP 4

Bake the meatballs in the preheated oven for about 12 minutes, or until browned all over but still moist.

STEP 5

While the meatballs are cooking, combine all the sauce ingredients in a dipping bowl and stir well.

STEP 6

Once the meatballs are cooked, transfer them to an airtight container and allow to cool slightly before sealing. Store the dipping sauce in a separate airtight container.

STEP 7

Refrigerate the meatballs and sauce for up to 3 days, or freeze for up to 3 weeks. Reheat before serving.

Cooking Difficulty:	Cooking Time:	Servings:
3/10	22 minutes	5

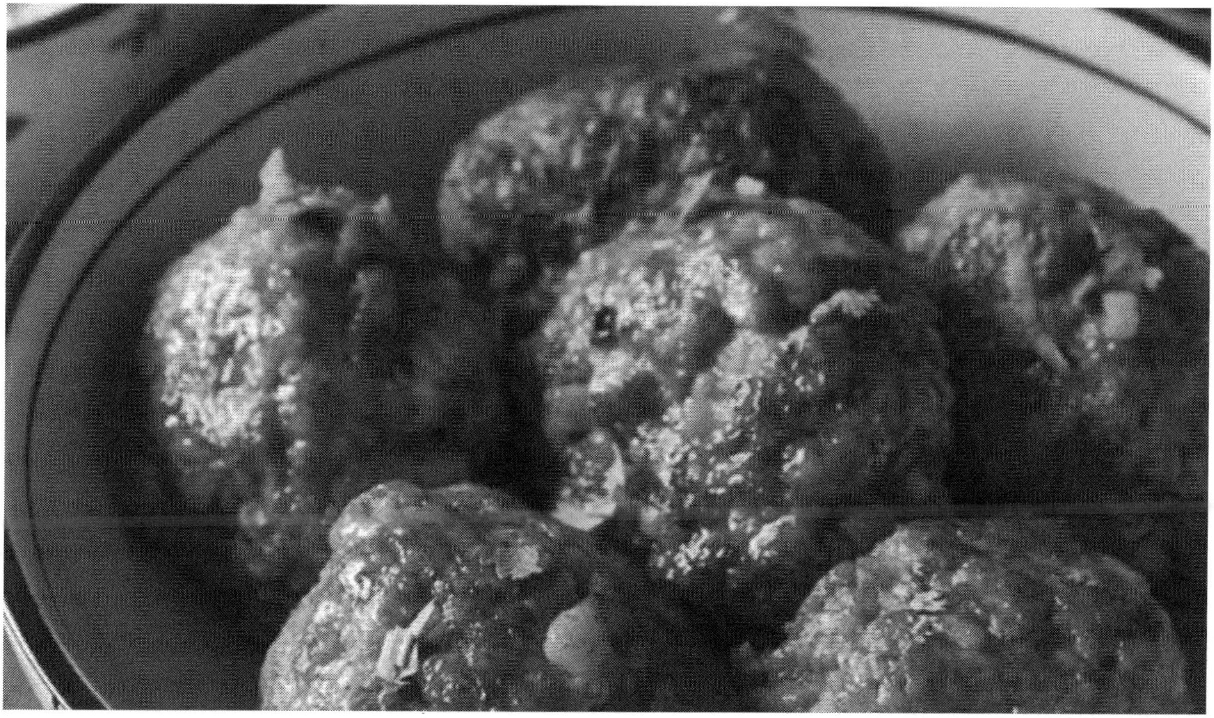

INGREDIENTS

- 1 lb. organic ground beef
- 1 large egg
- 1 minced red onion
- 2 minced garlic cloves
- ½ tsp. sea salt
- black pepper
- for the sauce:
- 1 minced garlic clove
- ¼ c. light soy sauce
- 2 tbsps. rice wine vinegar
- 1 tbsps. grated ginger
- 1 tbsp. chopped green onion
- liquid stevia
- nonstick cooking spray

NUTRITIONAL INFORMATION

238 Calories, 14g Fats, 3g Net Carbs, 24g Protein

BALSAMIC HERBED PORK TENDERLOIN

STEP 1

Set the oven to 475 degrees F to preheat.

STEP 2

Blot the pork medallions dry with paper towels then season with salt and pepper.

STEP 3

Place an ovenproof skillet over medium-high flame and heat through. Once hot, add the olive oil and ¾ tablespoon of butter then swirl to coat.

STEP 4

Add the garlic and shallot, then sauté until fragrant. Add the pork medallions and sear for 2 minutes per side.

STEP 5

Stir in the balsamic vinegar, soy sauce, thyme, rosemary, and remaining butter. Stir well to combine, then spoon the mixture over the pork.

STEP 6

Simmer for 2 minutes, then bake for 5 minutes.

STEP 7

After 5 minutes, turn over the pork medallions and cook for an added 5 minutes, or until the internal temperature of the pork is 150 degrees F.

STEP 8

Transfer the pork to a platter and let rest for 3 minutes. Then, divide into individual servings and spoon the sauce on top. Cover and refrigerate for up to 3 days.

Cooking Difficulty: 4/10	Cooking Time: 32 minutes	Servings: 2

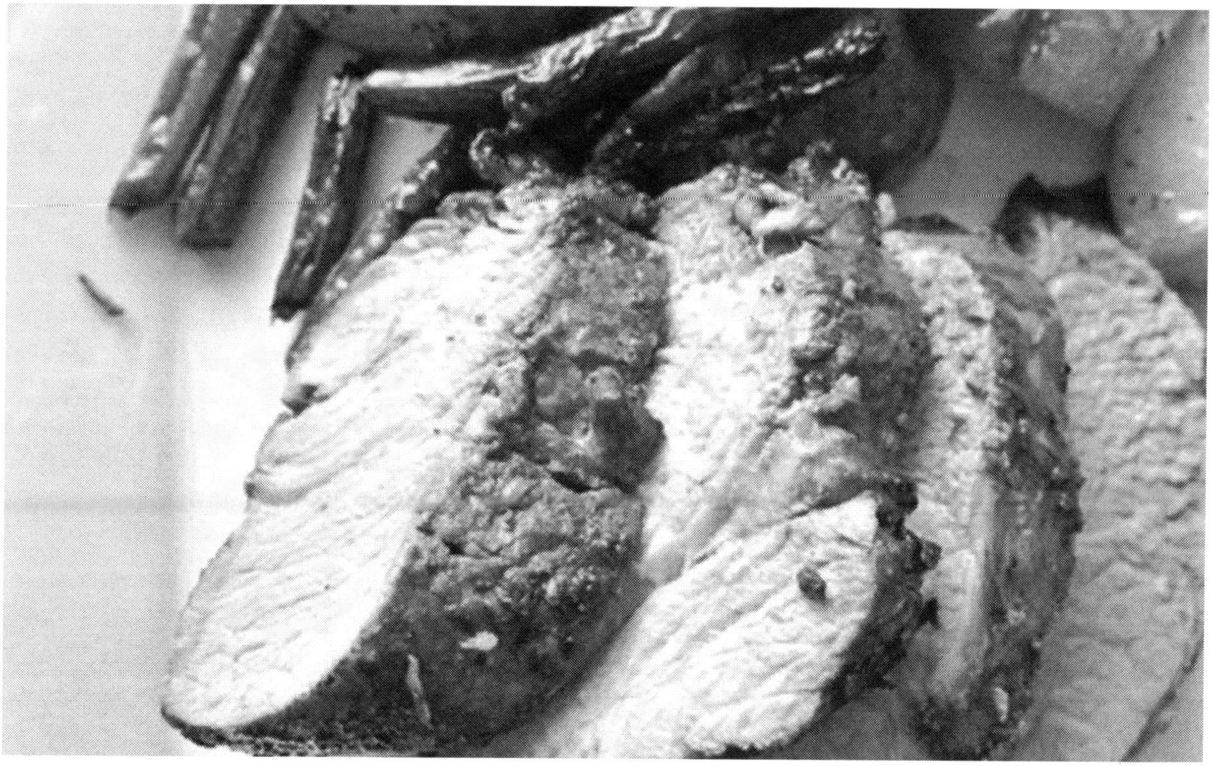

INGREDIENTS

- ¾ lb. pork tenderloin
- 1 minced garlic clove
- 1 minced shallot
- 3 tbsps. butter
- 2 tbsps. balsamic vinegar
- 1½ tbsps. olive oil
- ¾ tsp. soy sauce
- 3 fresh rosemary sprigs
- 3 fresh thyme sprigs
- sea salt
- black pepper

NUTRITIONAL INFORMATION

508 Calories, 34g Fats, 4g Net Carbs, 45g Protein

SARDINE AND GARDEN SALAD

Cooking Difficulty: 2/10	Cooking Time: 5 minutes	Servings: 3

INGREDIENTS

- 1 diced cucumber
- 2 diced tomatoes
- 1 minced red onion
- 2 chopped sardine fillets
- 2 c. chopped arugula leaves
- ¼ c. chopped fresh flat-leaf parsley

for the dressing:

- 2 tbsps. extra virgin olive oil
- ½ tbsp. squeezed lemon juice
- sea salt
- black pepper

STEP 1

Combine the ingredients for the dressing in a bowl and set aside.

STEP 2

Toss together the chopped sardines, vegetables, and herbs in a bowl. Mix well, then divide into individual servings.

STEP 3

Divide the whole sardine fillets among the servings.

STEP 4

Drizzle the dressing over the salads, then cover and refrigerate for up to 3 days.

NUTRITIONAL INFORMATION

150 Calories, 11g Fats, 8g Net Carbs, and 6g Protein

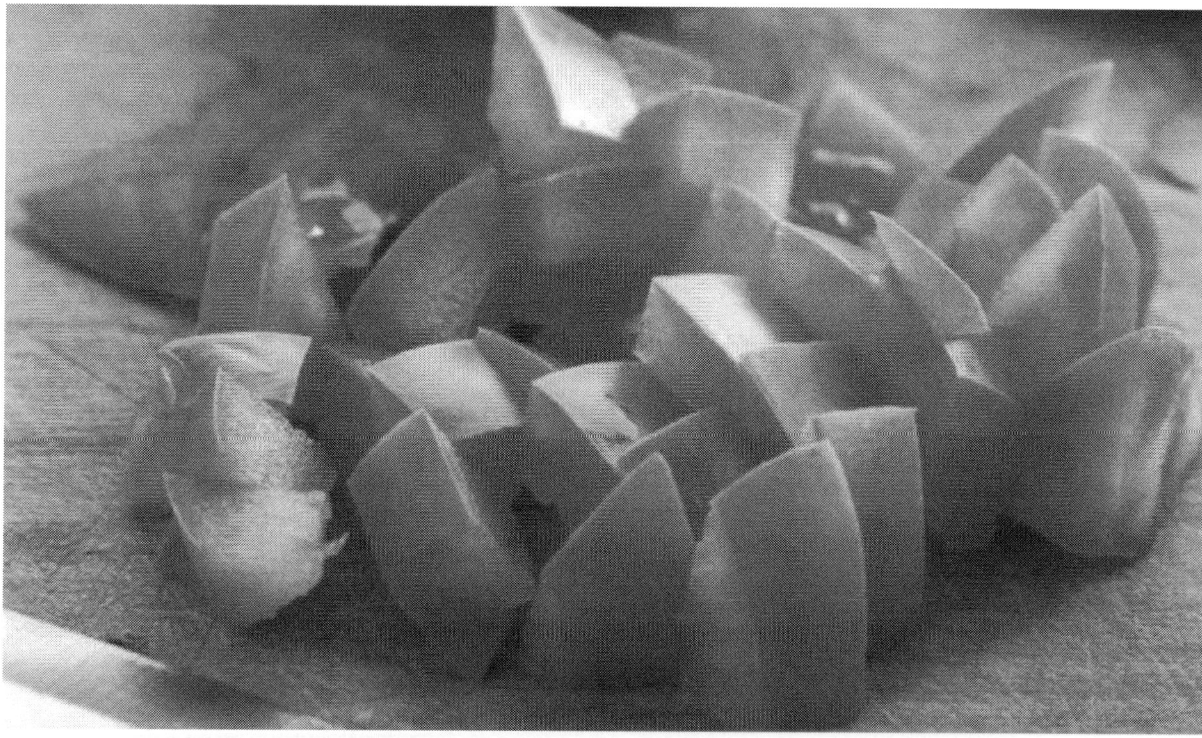

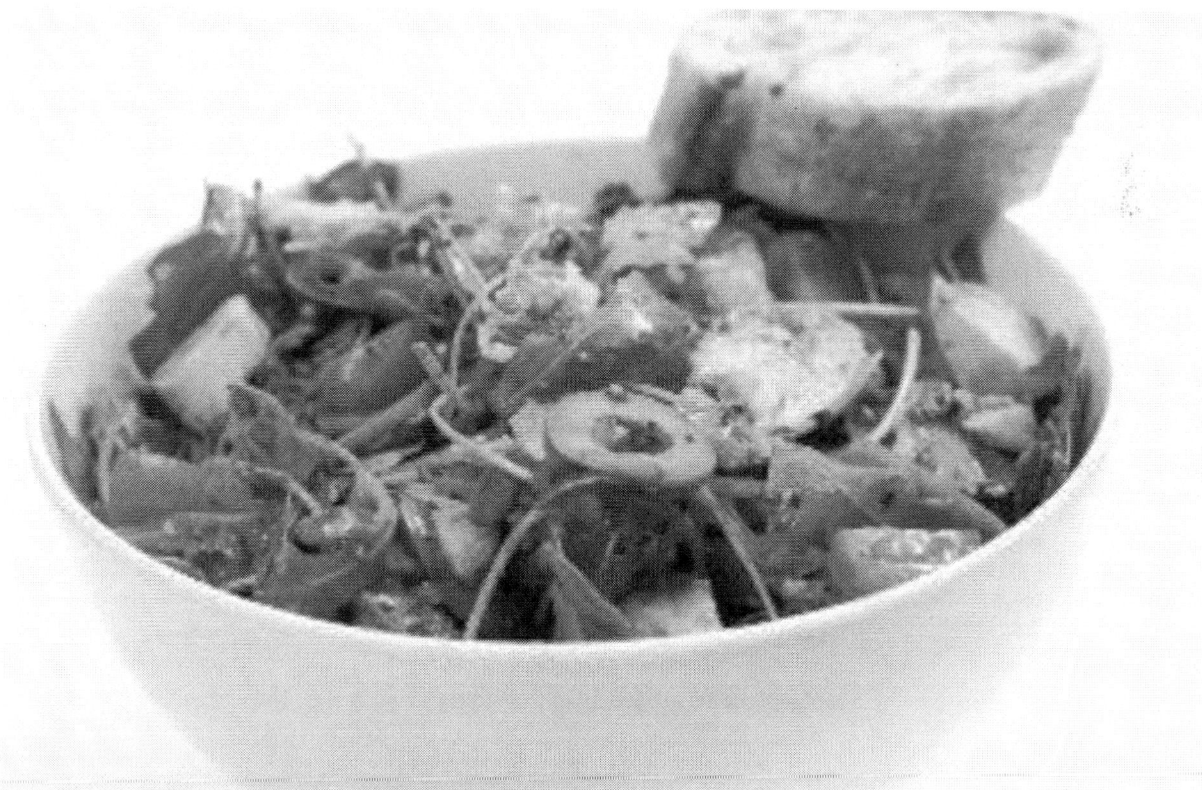

ZUCCHINI BEEF LASAGNA

Cooking Difficulty: 4/10	Cooking Time: 85 minutes	Servings: 10

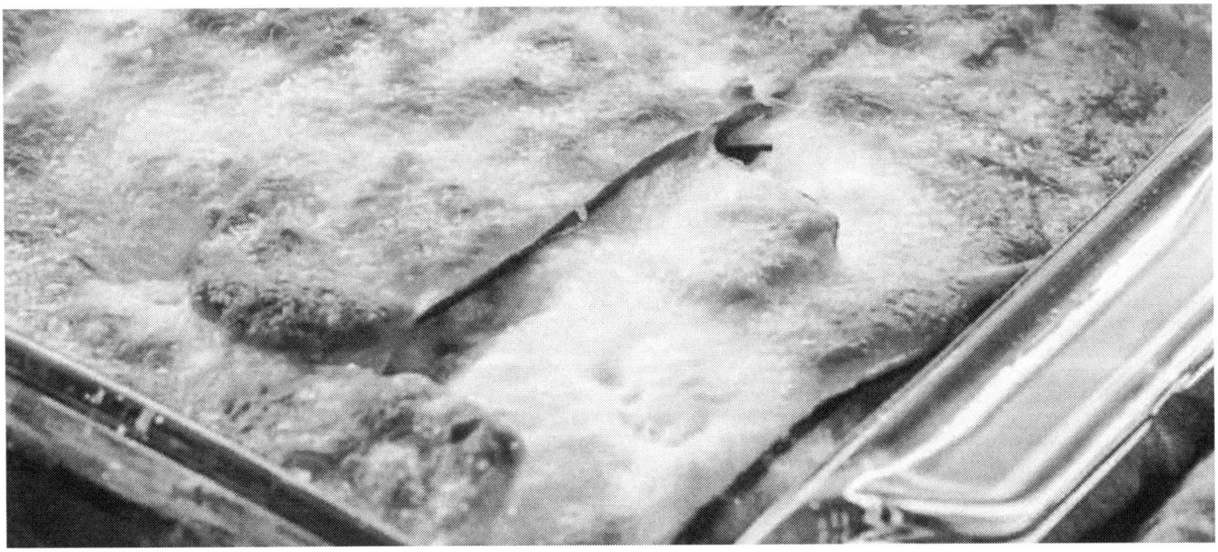

INGREDIENTS

- 2 large zucchinis
- 1 large yellow onion, chopped
- 2 minced garlic cloves
- 1 lb. 75 percent lean ground beef
- 2 c. no sugar organic pasta sauce
- 1 c. ricotta cheese
- ½ c. shredded Parmesan cheese
- 8 tbsps. shredded mozzarella cheese
- 2 tbsps. chopped fresh oregano
- 2 tbsps. olive oil
- 1 tbsp. chopped fresh basil
- ¼ tsp. fine sea salt
- ¼ tsp. black pepper

NUTRITIONAL INFORMATION

366 Calories, 15g Fats, 12g Net Carbs, 46g Protein

STEP 1
Set the oven to 375 degrees F to preheat.

STEP 2
Place a saucepan over medium-high flame and heat through. Once hot, add the olive oil and swirl to coat.

STEP 3
Sauté the onion in the saucepan until tender, then stir in the garlic and sauté until fragrant.

STEP 4
Add the ground beef to the saucepan and stir, breaking up, until browned all over.

STEP 5
Stir in the pasta sauce, then bring to a simmer. Once simmering, reduce to low flame and stir in the basil, oregano, and salt. Mix well, then set aside.

STEP 6
Halve the zucchinis lengthwise, then slice into extra thin strips, about 1/8 inch thick.

STEP 7
Arrange 6 zucchini slices on the bottom of the baking dish, then add a quarter of the meat sauce on top. Add ¼ cup of ricotta cheese with 2 tablespoons of mozzarella cheese. Repeat, ensuring the zucchini slices crisscross.

STEP 8
Once the lasagna is assembled, top with Parmesan cheese and black pepper. Bake in the oven for 1 hour, or until the top is browned and bubbling.

STEP 9
Carefully remove the lasagna from the oven and place on the kitchen counter. Allow to sit for about 15 minutes, then slice into 10 equal servings. Allow to cool slightly, then cover and refrigerate for up to 4 days. Reheat before serving.

BAKED CHICKEN NUGGETS

Cooking Difficulty: 3/10	Cooking Time: 38 minutes	Servings: 4

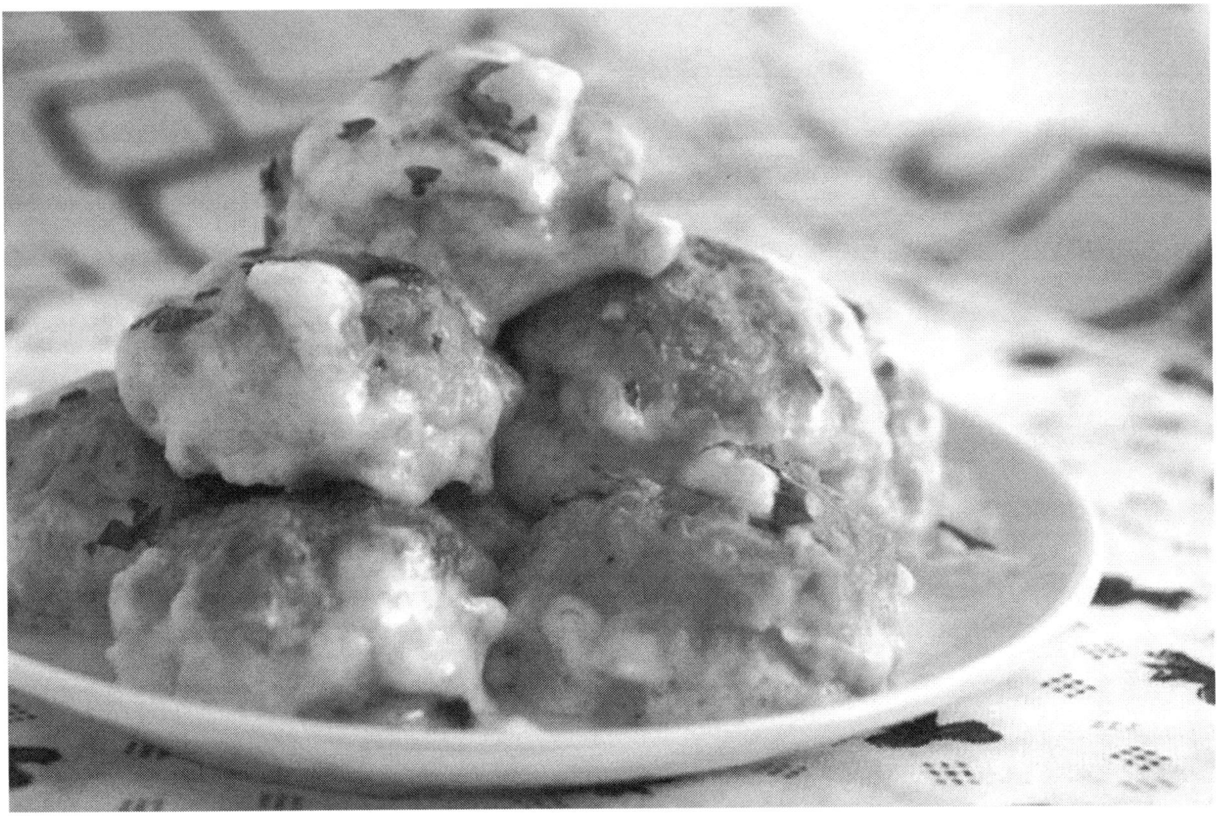

NUTRITIONAL INFORMATION

282 Calories, 12g Fats, 11g Net Carbs, 33g Protein

INGREDIENTS

- ½ tsp. dried oregano
- 1 tsp. salt
- ½ c. parmesan cheese
- ½ c. milk
- 1 c. marinara sauce
- 1 c. almond flour
- 3 oz. mozzarella cheese
- 1 lb. minced chicken breast

STEP 1

Allow the oven to heat up to 350 degrees. Coat a baking dish and set to the side.

STEP 2

Combine half the almond flour with the pepper, salt, cheese, and milk in a bowl. Add in the chicken and mix to combine.

STEP 3

Divide this into 24 balls and then dredge through the reserved almond flour.

STEP 4

Place onto the baking dish and place into the oven. Bake for a total of 20 minutes but flip around halfway through.

STEP 5

Once these are done, pour the sauce on top and then dot with some cheese. Place back in the oven.

STEP 6

After 15 minutes, take this out of the oven and serve.

CHICKEN BACON WRAPS

Cooking Difficulty: 3/10	Cooking Time: 48 minutes	Servings: 8

INGREDIENTS

- 12 skinless and boneless chicken breast halves
- 12 slices of bacon
- 16 oz. chive and onion cream cheese
- 12 tbsps. divided olive oil spread
- salt

STEP 1

Flatten the chicken breasts to 1/2-inch thickness.

STEP 2

Spread 3 tablespoons of cream cheese over each chicken breast.

STEP 3

Dot with 1 tablespoon olive oil spread and sprinkle with the salt; roll up and wrap each rolled piece with a bacon strip.

STEP 4

Grease your pan and place chicken onto it and bake uncovered for about 40 minutes at 400 degrees F or until the juices run clear.

STEP 5

Transfer the pan 6 inches from the heat source; broil for 5 minutes until the bacon is crispy.

NUTRITIONAL INFORMATION

502 Calories, 38.2 g Fat, 1.1 g Carbs, 38.1 g Protein

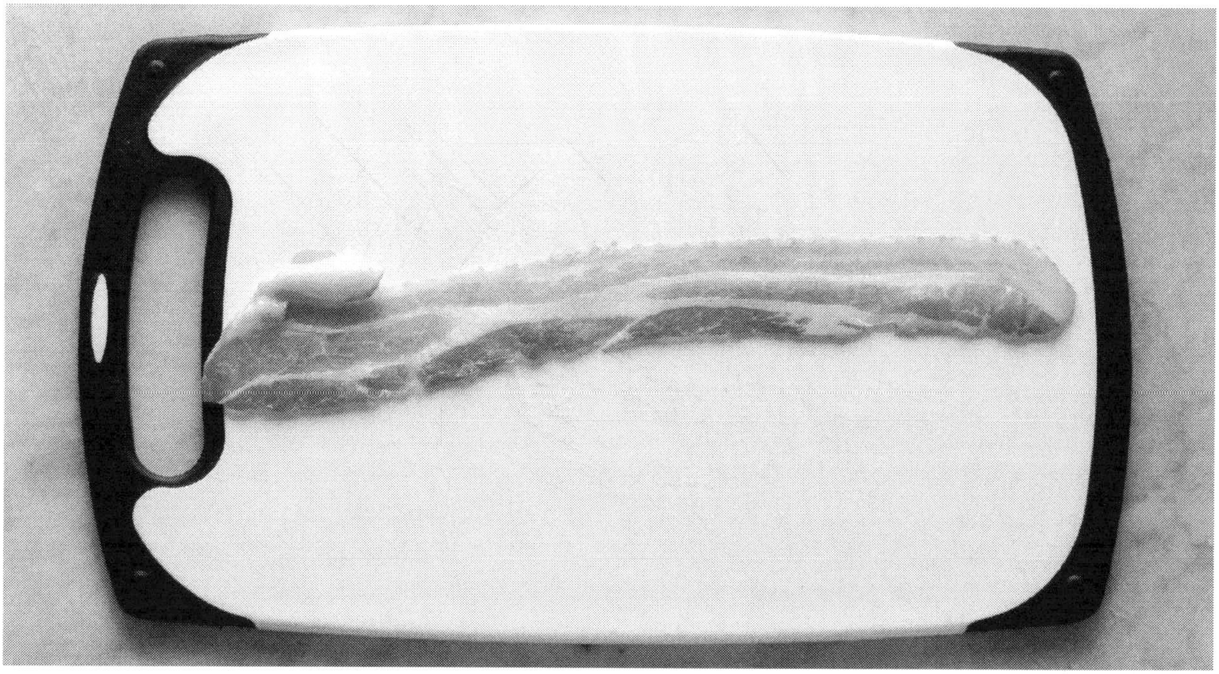

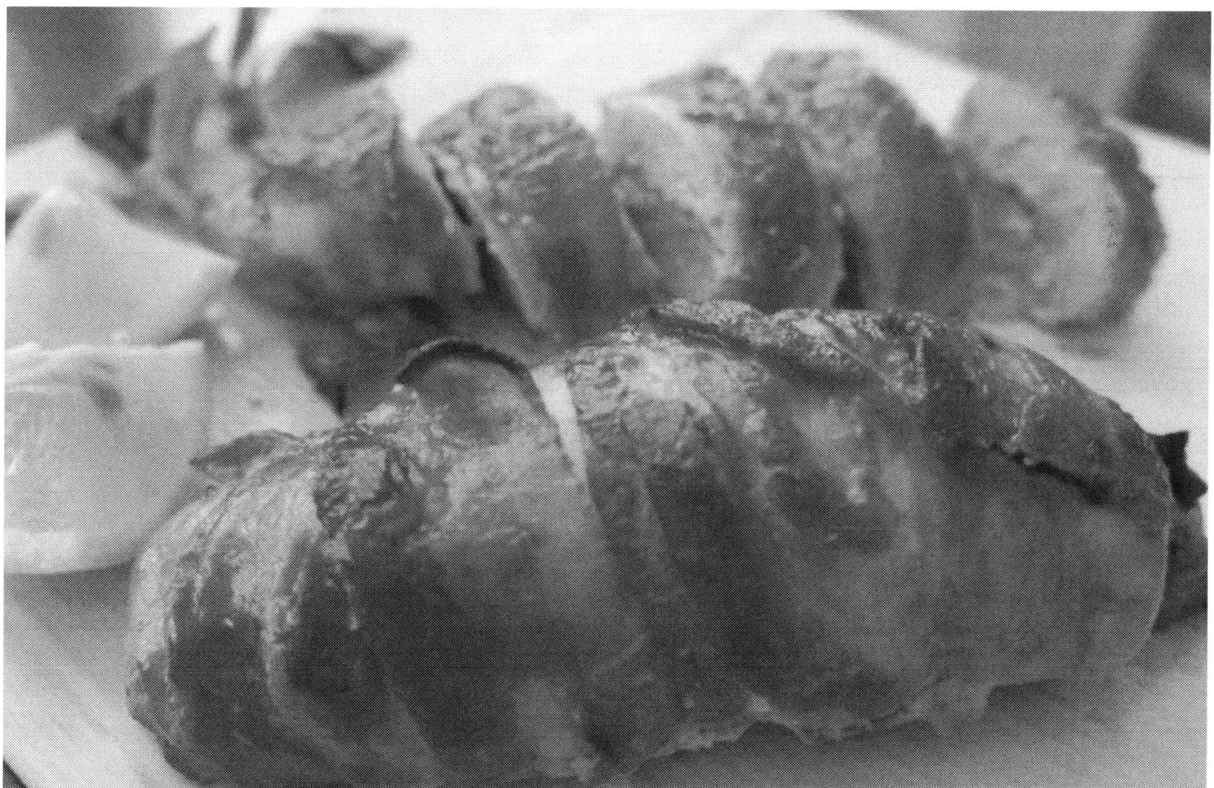

PORK SALAD

Cooking Difficulty: 3/10	Cooking Time: 35 minutes	Servings: 2

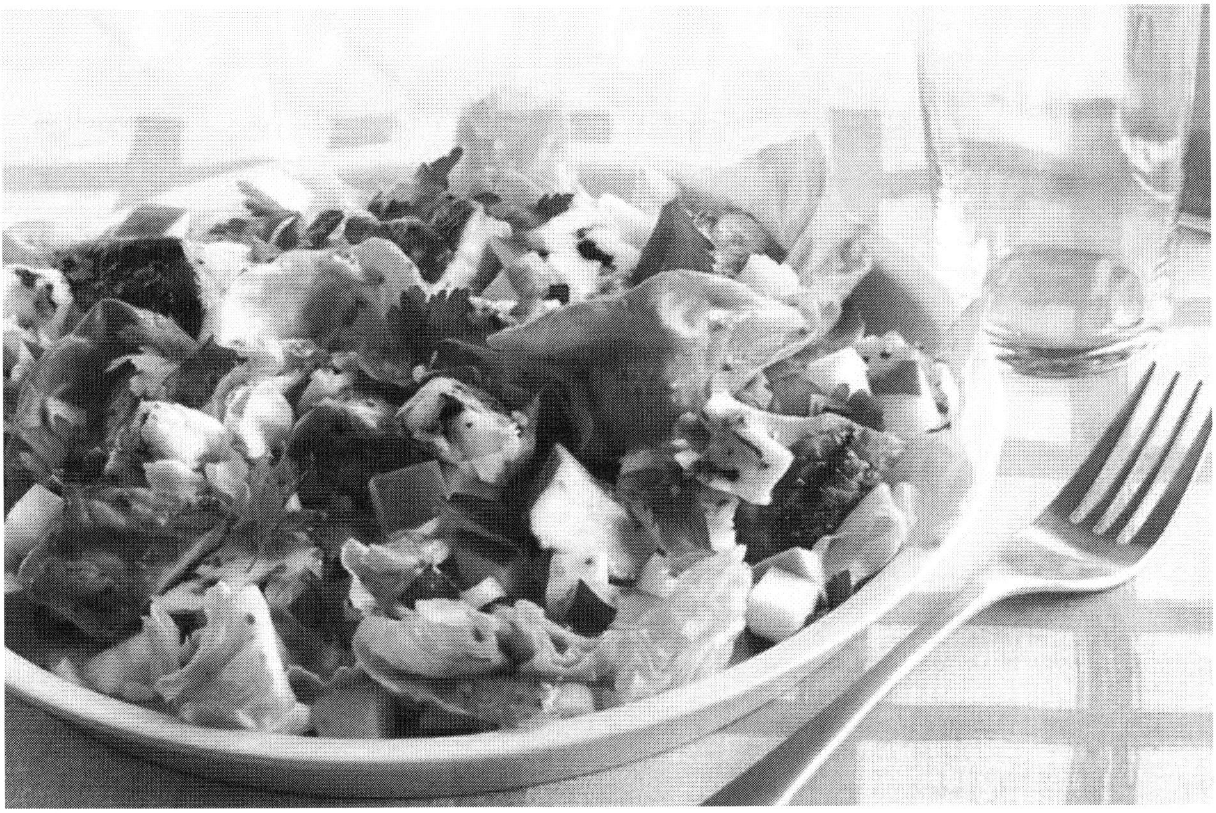

NUTRITIONAL INFORMATION

1050 Calories, 55g Fats, 5g Net Carbs, 13g Protein

INGREDIENTS

- ½ sliced pear
- 1/3 c. blue cheese
- ½ lb. pork belly slices
- 2 tsps. olive oil
- 2 tbsps. white wine vinegar
- ½ tsp. mustard
- 1 tsp. water
- 1 tbsp. stevia
- 1/3 c. chopped walnuts
- 2 tsps. salt
- 2 c. salad leaves

STEP 1

Cover the pork with half your oil and then cook it in the oven for 30 minutes.

STEP 2

Warm-up a pan and add the stevia and water. When the stevia dissolves, add the walnuts and cook for about five minutes.

STEP 3

Take the nuts and allow them to cool. While those are cooling, chop the cheese and pear into smaller bits.

STEP 4

To make the dressing, add the oil, vinegar, and mustard to a bowl.

STEP 5

Take the pork out of the oven and slice into smaller bits. Toss the salad with the dressing before adding the rest of the ingredients and serving.

VEGETABLE WRAPS

Cooking Difficulty: 2/10	Cooking Time: 9 minutes	Servings: 4

INGREDIENTS

- 1 head of romaine lettuce
- 2 carrots
- 1 cucumber
- 1 red onion
- 1 celery stalk
- dressing of choice

STEP 1

Finely slice the carrots, cucumber, red onion, and celery into sticks of vegetable.

STEP 2

Divide between 12 lettuce leaves.

STEP 3

Roll up lettuce leaves and serve.

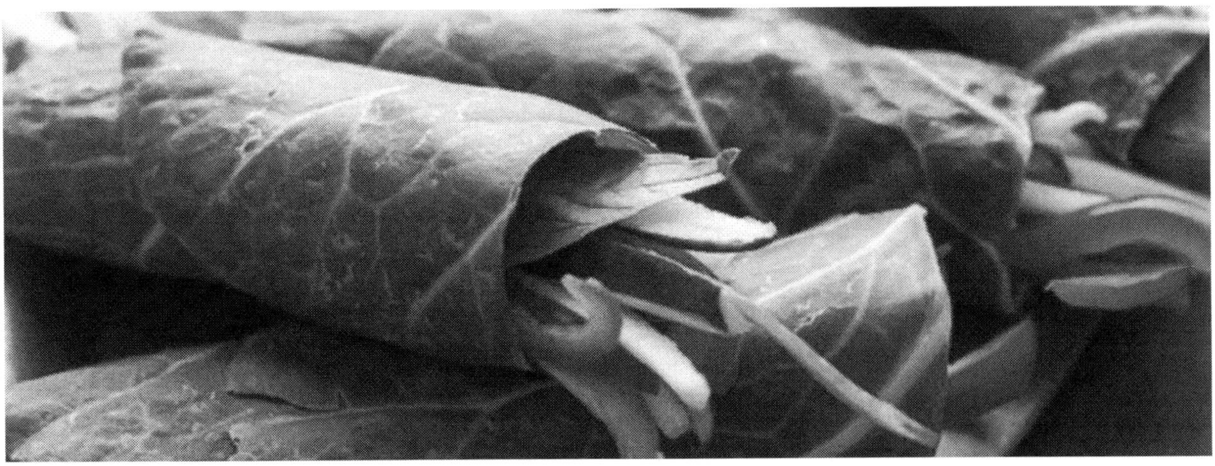

NUTRITIONAL INFORMATION

20 Calories, 0g Fats, 5g Net Carbs, and 0g Protein

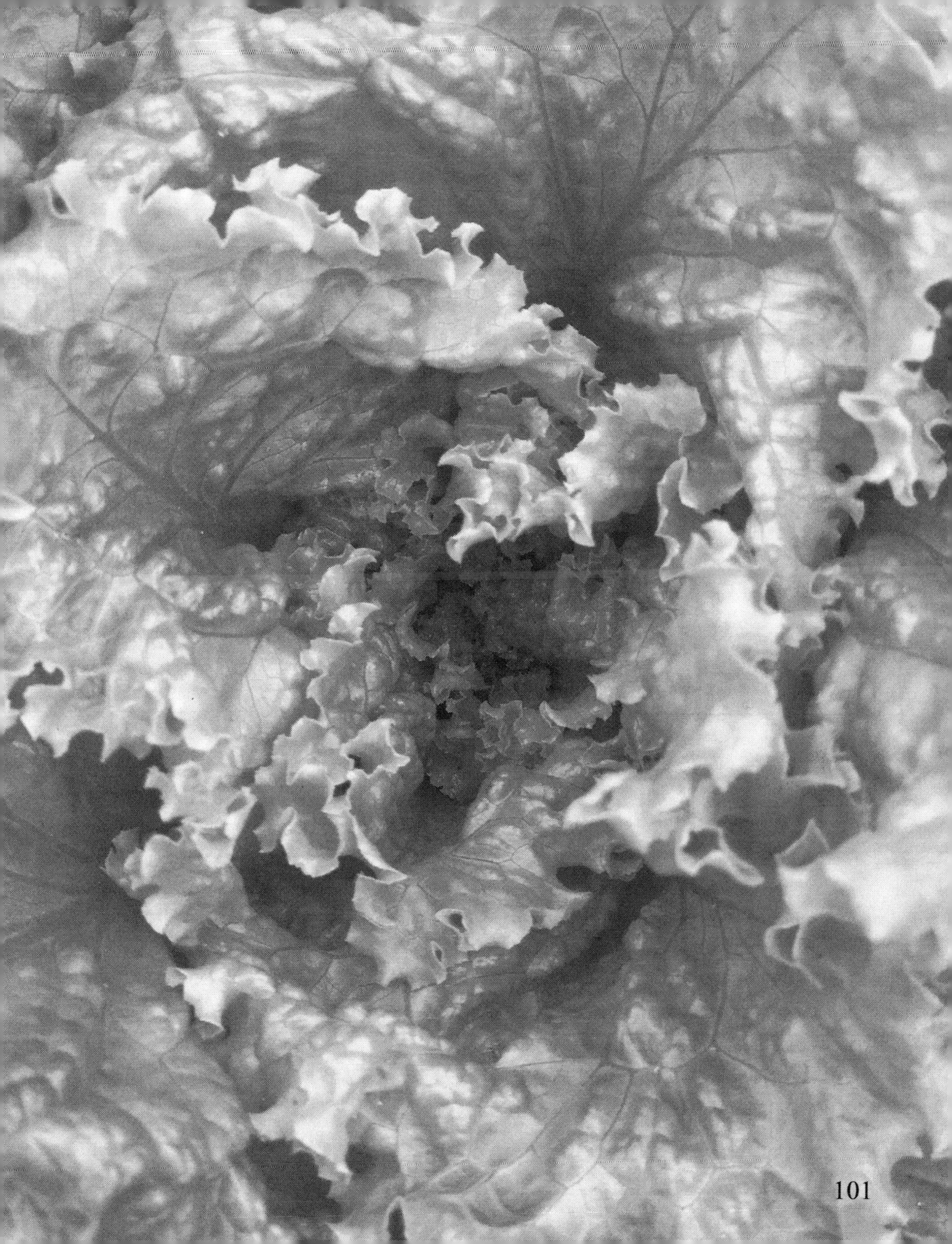

KETO PORK AND PLUMS

Cooking Difficulty: 3/10	Cooking Time: 240 minutes	Servings: 8

INGREDIENTS

- 2 lb. pork belly
- 4 chopped plums
- 1 c. bouillon
- 1 tbsp. allspice
- 1 tbsp. cinnamon

STEP 1

Make slices in the skin of the pork, so the flavor of the plums soaks through.

STEP 2

Rub with allspice and cinnamon.

STEP 3

Mix remaining ingredients into a sauce.

STEP 4

Place pork in the pot. Stew for four hours.

NUTRITIONAL INFORMATION

316Calories, 20g Fats, 10g Net Carbs, 24g Protein

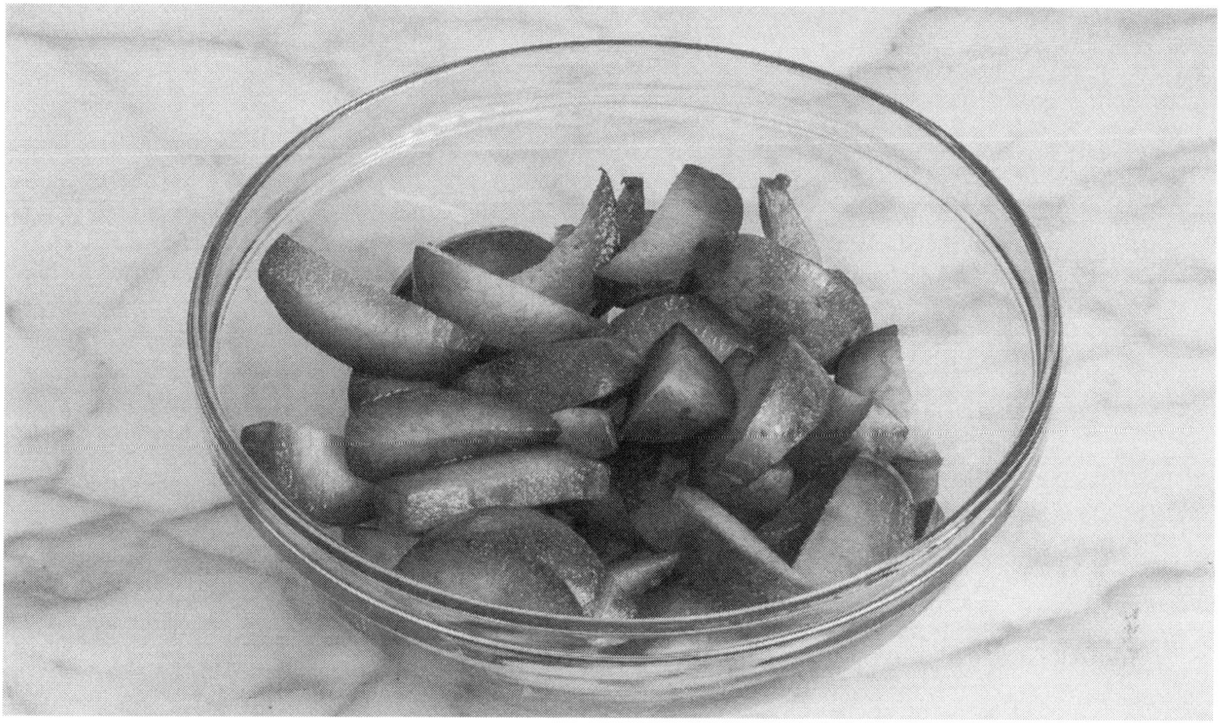

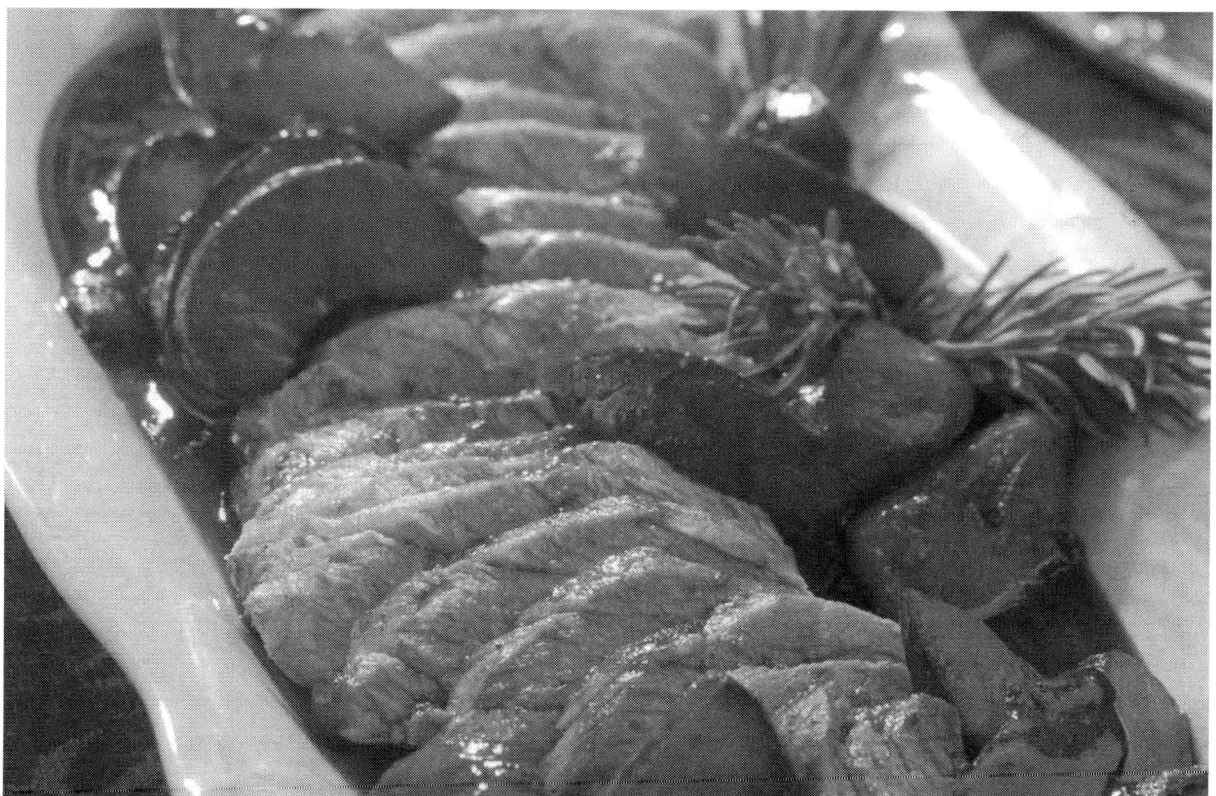

DINNER RECIPES

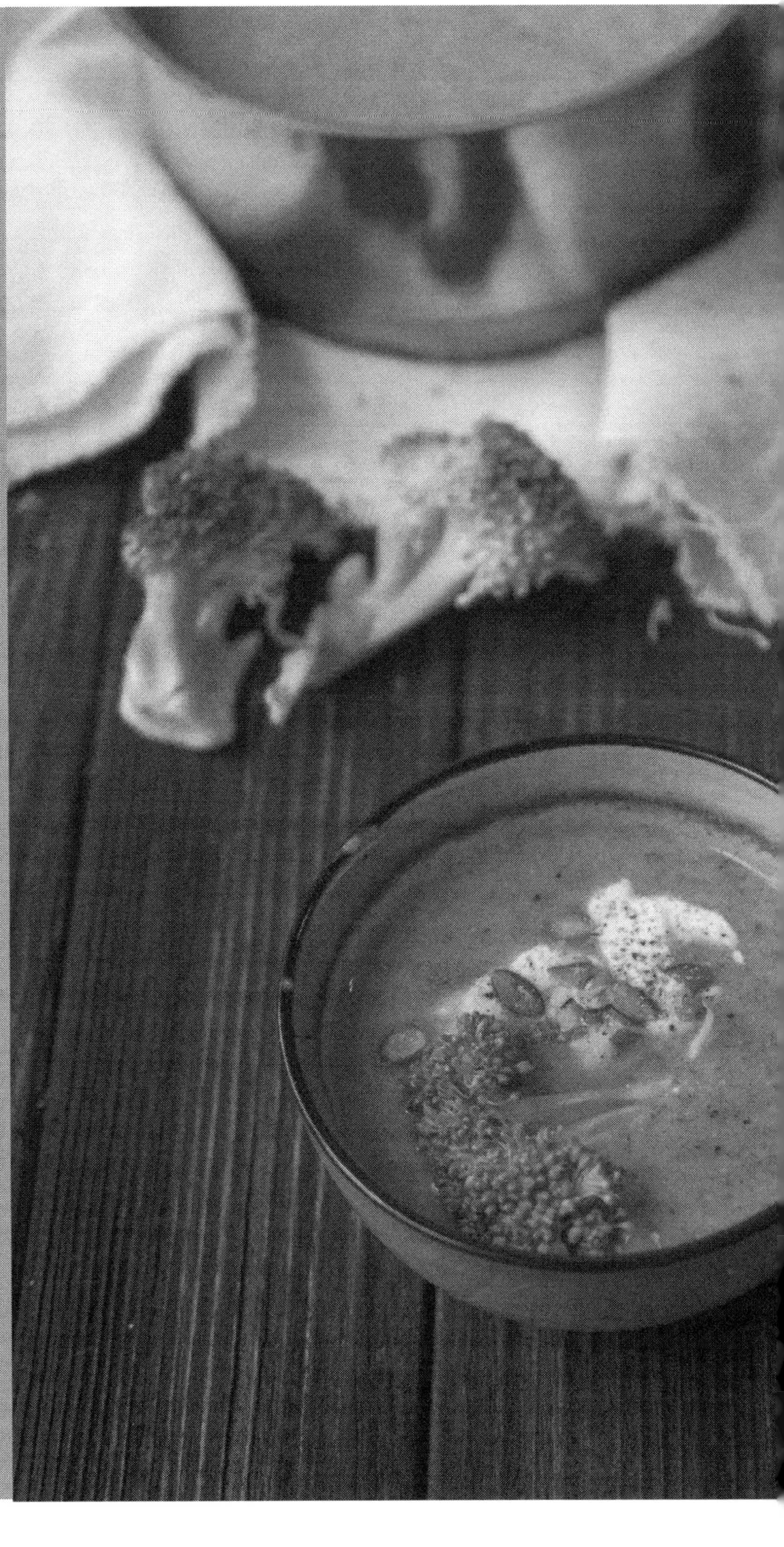

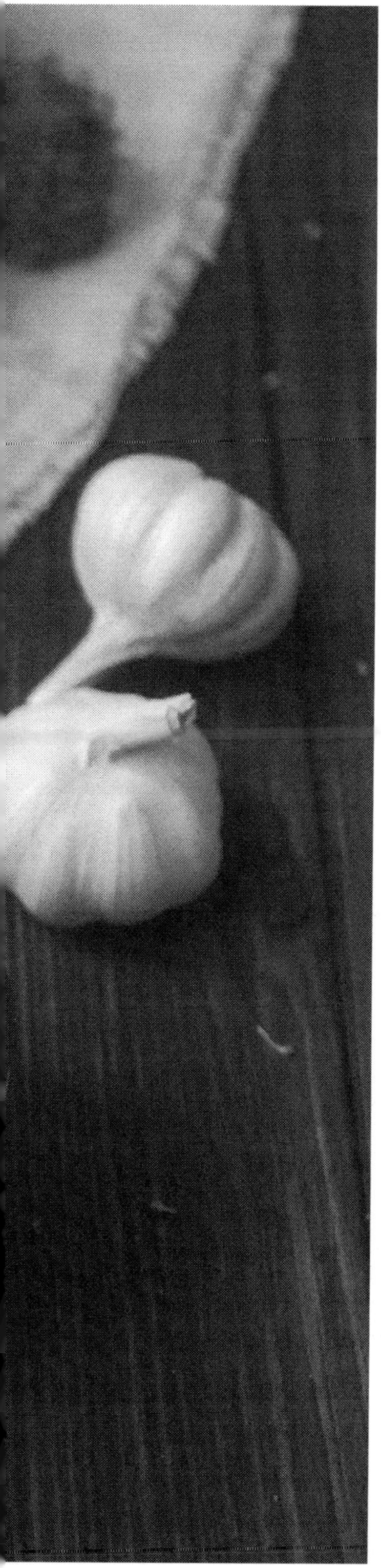

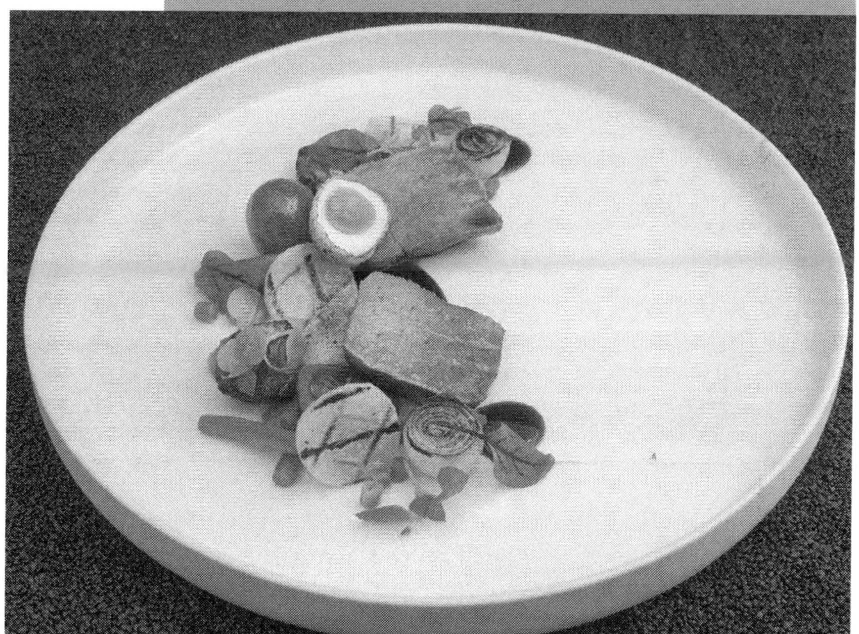

SIMPLE BEEF CHILI

Cooking Difficulty: 4/10	Cooking Time: 65 minutes	Servings: 3

INGREDIENTS

- 1 diced yellow onion
- 1 lb. ground beef
- 2 c. organic beef broth
- ¼ c. extra virgin olive oil
- 2 tbsps. flaxseed meal
- 1 tbsp. chili powder
- 1 tsp. dried oregano
- ½ tsp. cumin seeds
- ¼ tsp. garlic powder
- sea salt
- black pepper

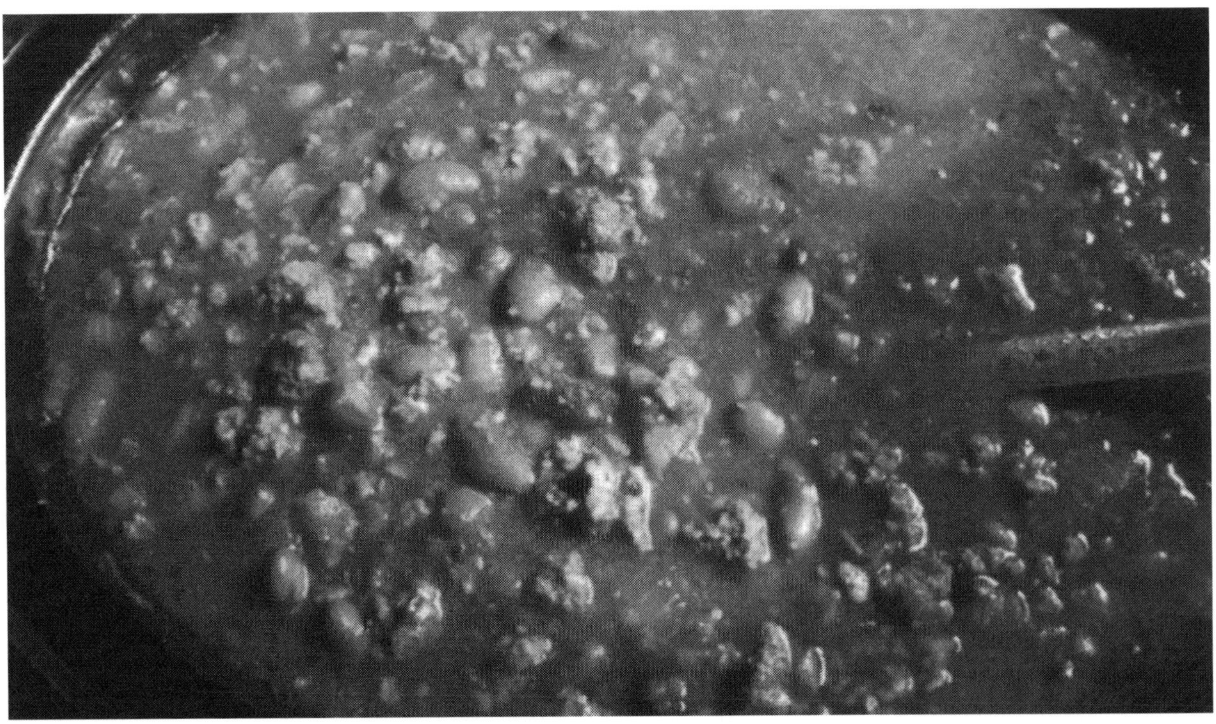

NUTRITIONAL INFORMATION

567 Calories, 36g Fats, 18g Net Carbs, 41g Protein

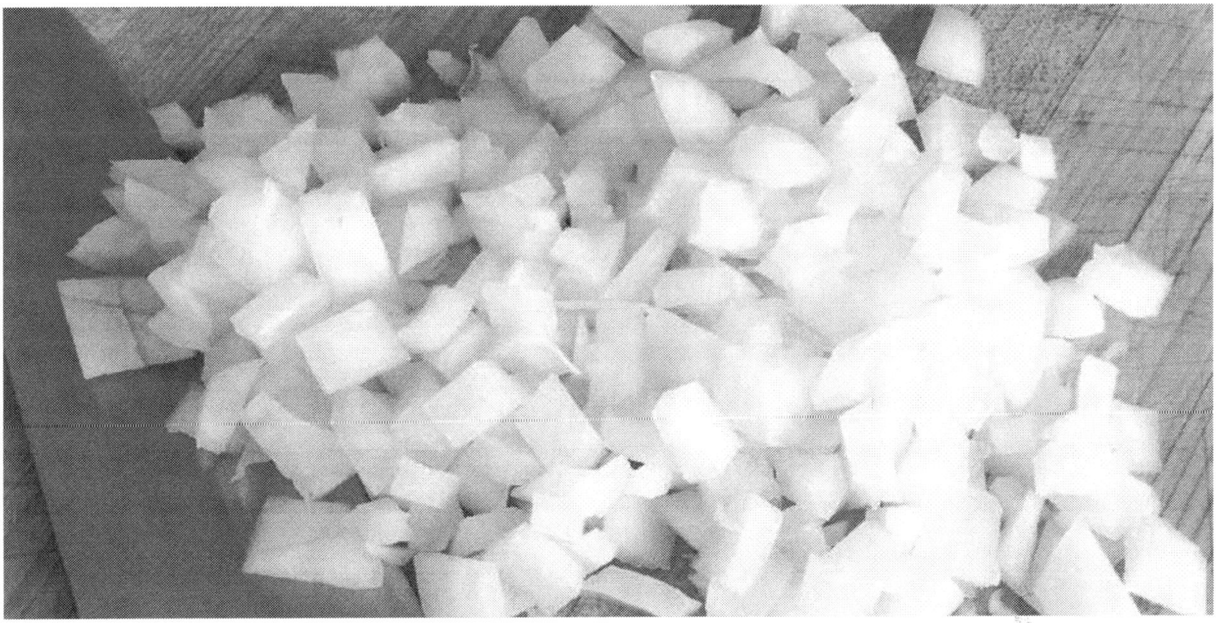

STEP 1

Place a heavy-duty pot over high flame and heat through. Once hot, add the beef and onion and sauté until the beef is browned.

STEP 2

Stir in the chili powder, oregano, cumin seeds, and garlic powder, then sauté until combined.

STEP 3

Pour in the beef broth, flaxseed meal, and olive oil. Stir to combine, then bring to a boil.

STEP 4

Once boiling, reduce to medium-high flame and simmer, partially covered, for 1 hour or until the chili is thickened.

STEP 5

Remove from heat and cover. Allow to cool, then transfer to airtight containers and refrigerate for up to 3 days. Reheat and season to taste with salt and pepper before serving.

SEA BASS

Cooking Difficulty: 2/10	Cooking Time: 18 minutes	Servings: 2

INGREDIENTS

- 2 lemons
- 1/3 c. green olives
- 1 c. grated cauliflower
- 1 seabass
- pepper
- salt
- 1/3 c. chopped parsley
- 1/3 c. chopped mint

STEP 1

Allow the oven to heat up to 400 degrees. Place some parchment paper on a baking pan and place the fish on top. Add some oil to the fish.

STEP 2

Slice the lemons and stuff them into the bass along with the herbs. Place into the oven to bake for 15 minutes.

STEP 3

Chop up the olives and juice the other lemons. Take out a bowl and mix together the rest of the ingredients.

STEP 4

Serve the prepared fish with the cauliflower salad.

NUTRITIONAL INFORMATION

380 Calories, 26g Fats, 3.4g Net Carbs, 27g Protein

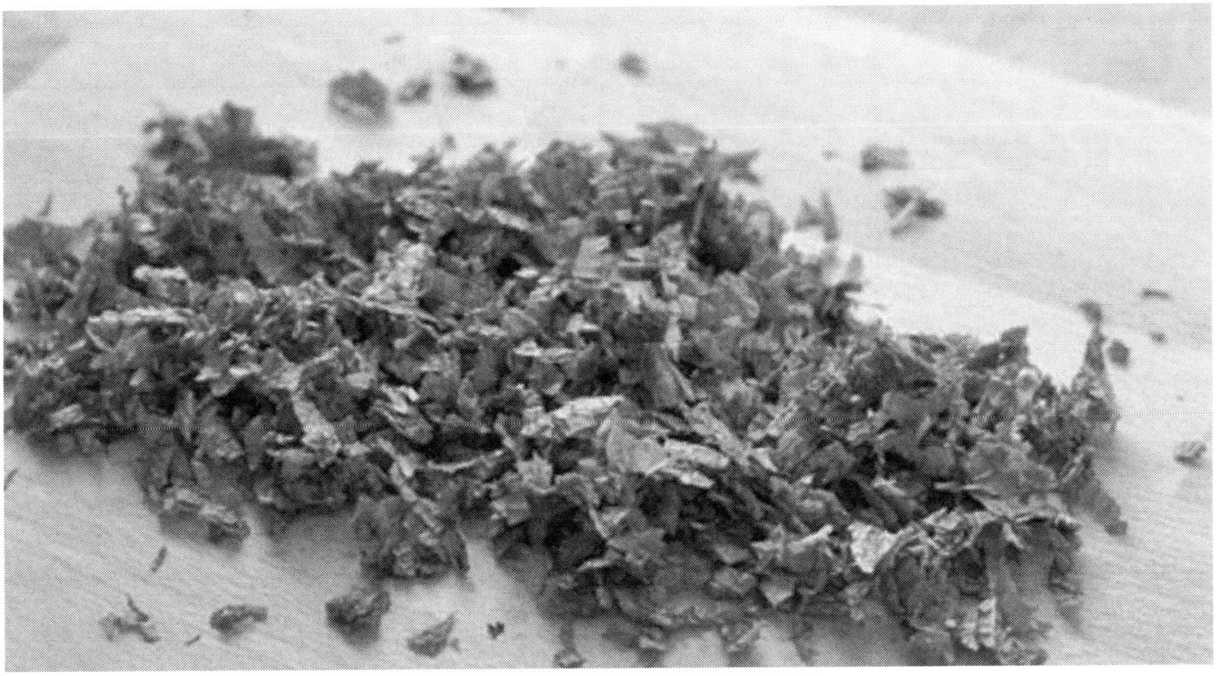

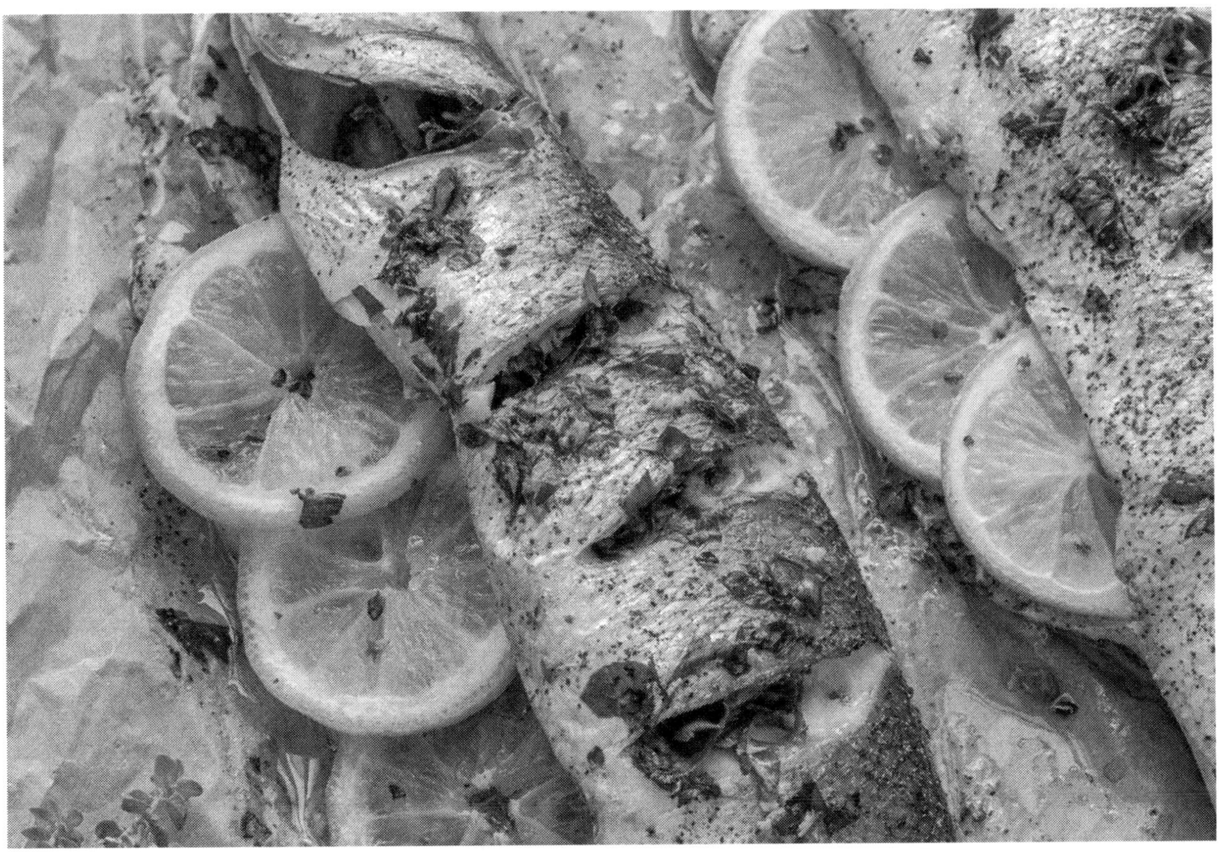

LOW CARB HEARTY POT ROAST

Cooking Difficulty: 5/10	Cooking Time: 280 minutes	Servings: 3

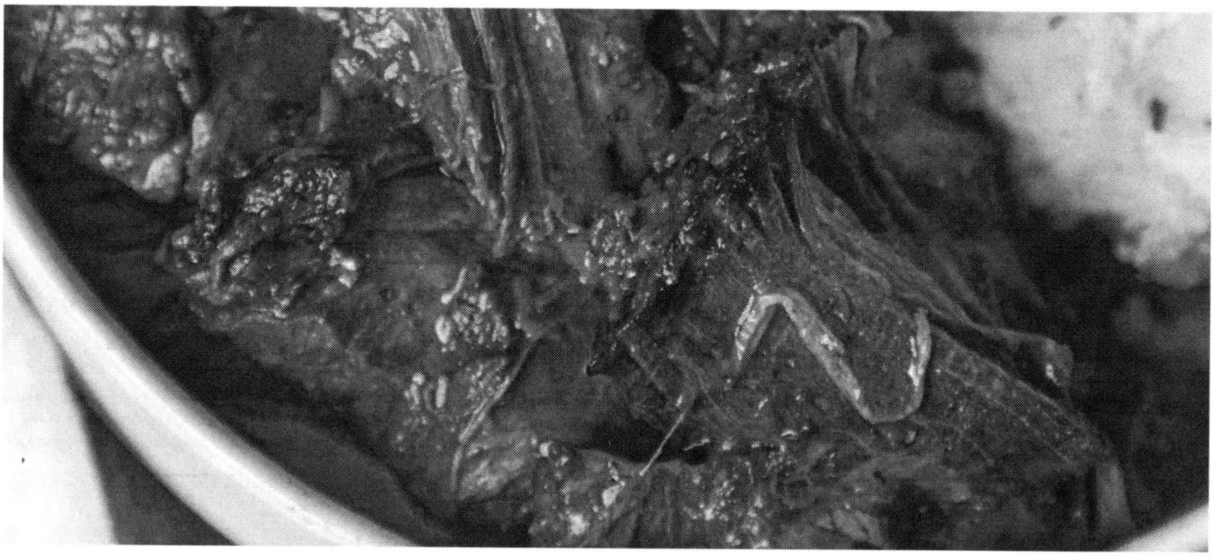

INGREDIENTS

- 2½ lb. bottom round rump roast
- 1 small onion
- 1 large garlic clove
- 1 fresh thyme sprig
- 1 chopped turnip
- 1½ c. beef stock
- 1 c. halved radishes
- 2 tbsps. heavy cream
- 1½ tbsps. olive oil
- sea salt
- black pepper

NUTRITIONAL INFORMATION

521 Calories, 25g Fats,6g Net Carbs, and 69g Protein

STEP 1

Set the oven to 475 degrees F.

STEP 2

Season the pork all over with salt and pepper.

STEP 3

Place a Dutch oven over a high flame and add the olive oil. Swirl to coat, then brown the roast all over and set aside.

STEP 4

Sauté the onion in the same pot until browned, then transfer to the bowl with the pot roast.

STEP 5

Add the beef stock, garlic, and thyme, then mix well. Return the roast and onion, then add the radishes and turnips.

STEP 6

Place the pot, uncovered, in the oven and set it to 400 degrees F. Cook for 4 to 5 hours, or until the internal temperature of the pot roast is 130 degrees F.

STEP 7

Take the roast out of the pot and let cool. Then, transfer the vegetables and roast them to a bowl.

STEP 8

Place a saucepan over medium flame and add the liquid from the Dutch oven. Stir in the heavy cream, then bring to a boil. Then, reduce to a simmer.

STEP 9

Slice the pot roast thinly, then divide into individual servings. Divide the vegetables and sauce as well, then let cool slightly. Cover and refrigerate for up to 3 days.

GINGER HALIBUT

Cooking Difficulty: 2/10	Cooking Time: 18 minutes	Servings: 3

INGREDIENTS

- 24 oz. Alaskan halibut fillets
- 1½ tbsps. minced fresh ginger
- 1½ tsps. soy sauce
- 1½ tsps. olive oil
- ¾ tsp. rice wine vinegar

STEP 1

Set the oven to 400 degrees F to preheat. Line a baking sheet with aluminum foil and set it aside.

STEP 2

Combine rice vinegar and olive oils in a bowl, then stir in the soy sauce, and ginger.

STEP 3

Add the fish fillets and turn several times to coat.

STEP 4

Arrange the fish fillets on the prepared baking sheet—Bake for 17 minutes, or until done

STEP 5

Cover each fish fillet with aluminum foil and refrigerate for up to 3 days, or freeze for up to 2 weeks. Reheat before serving.

NUTRITIONAL INFORMATION

380 Calories, 26g Fats, 3.4g Net Carbs, 27g Protein

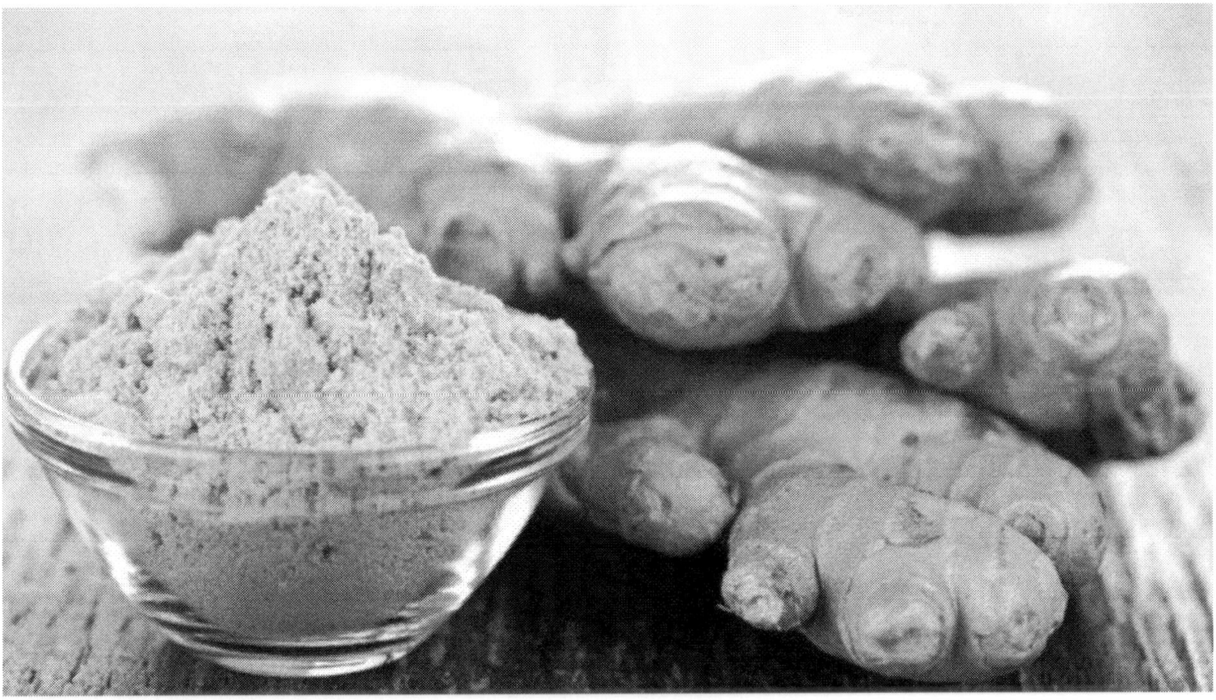

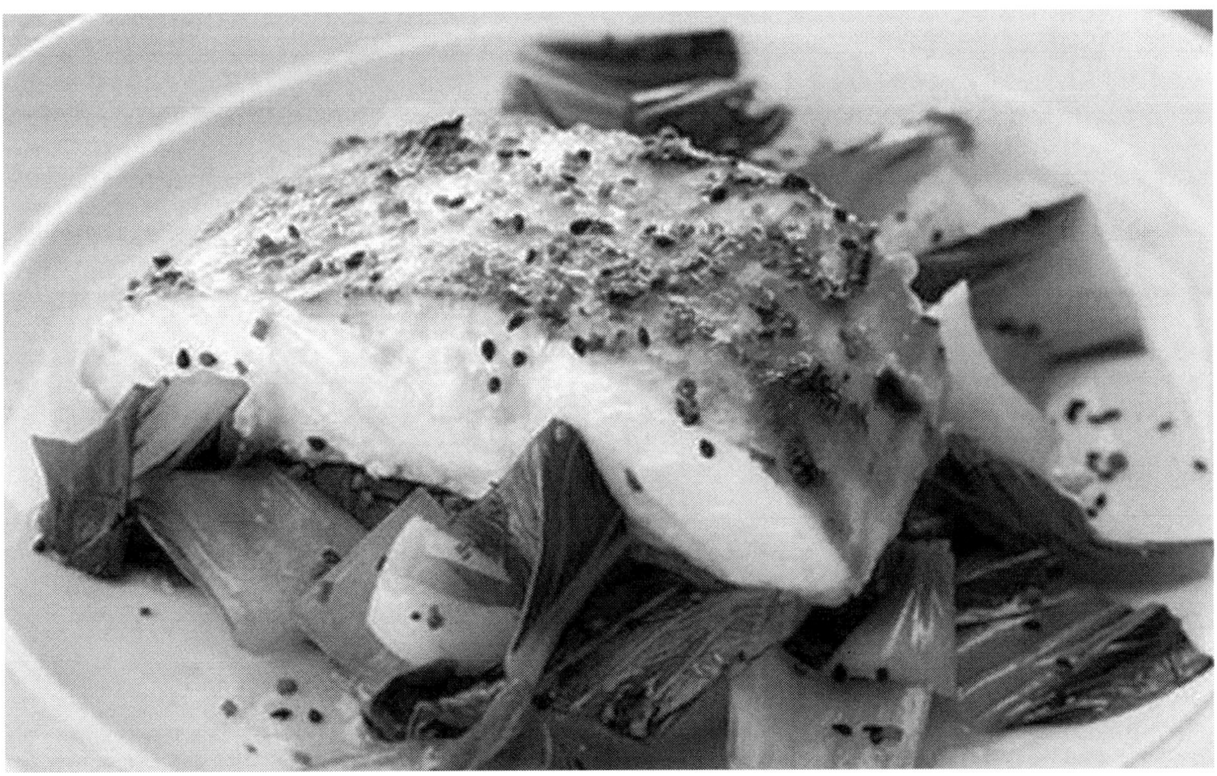

SUPER GREEN SOUP

Cooking Difficulty: 2/10	Cooking Time: 15 minutes	Servings: 6

INGREDIENTS

- pepper
- salt
- ¼ c. coconut oil
- 1 c. coconut milk
- 4 c. vegetable stock
- 2 c. spinach
- 1 c. watercress
- 1 bay leaf
- 2 minced garlic cloves
- 1 chopped onion
- 1 chopped cauliflower head

STEP 1

Grease up a pan with some oil and cook the garlic and onion. When those are browned, add the bay leaf and cauliflower and cook for another 5 minutes.

STEP 2

Add the spinach and watercress and cook for a bit to wilt. Pour in the vegetable stock and let this boil. Cook for another 8 minutes.

STEP 3

Add in the coconut milk and then remove it from the heat. Blend so this becomes smooth and creamy.

STEP 4

This can be frozen or left in the fridge for five days.

NUTRITIONAL INFORMATION

392 Calories, 38g Fats, 7g Net Carbs, and 5g Protein

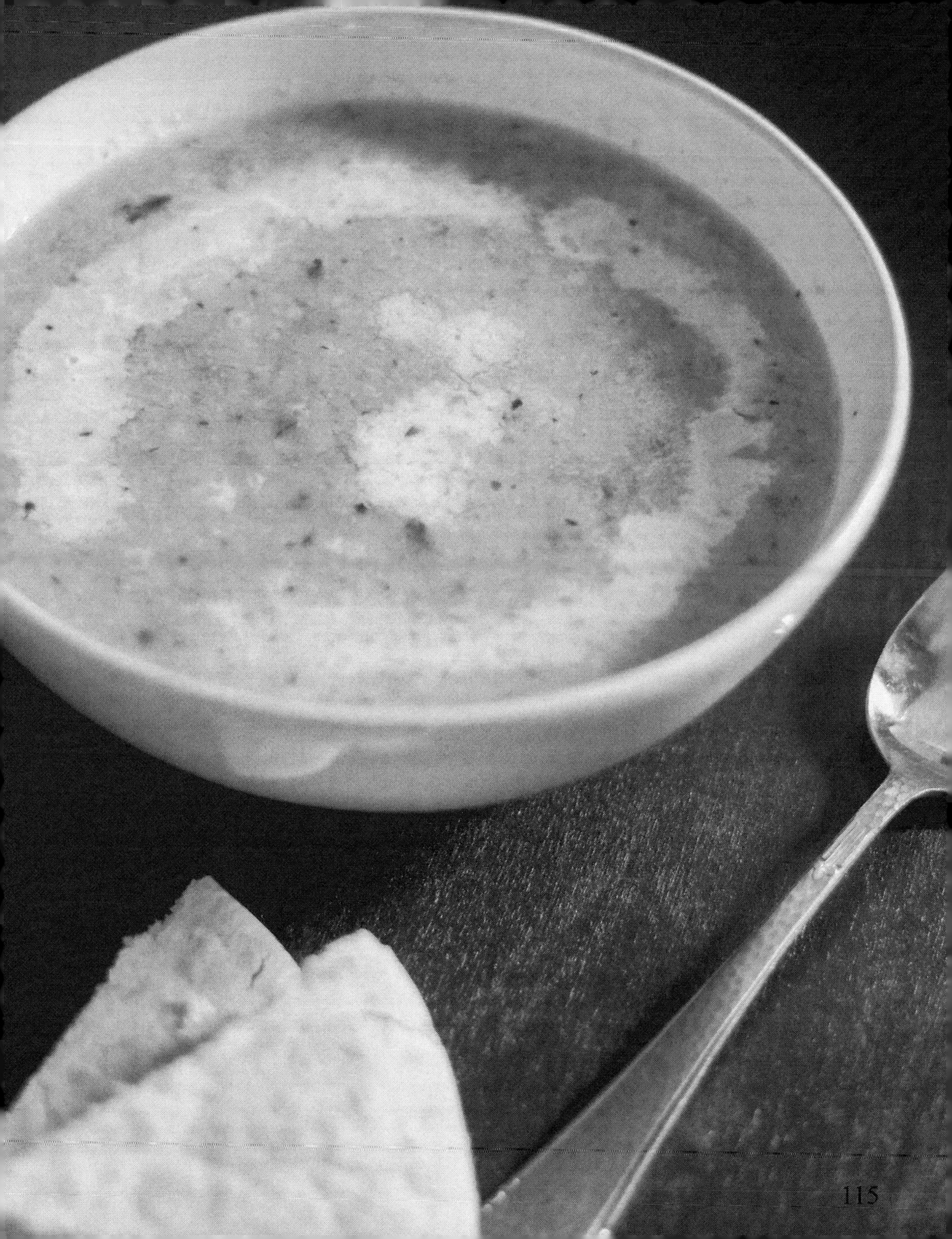

EGGS AND BACON

Cooking Difficulty: 2/10	Cooking Time: 23 minutes	Servings: 6

INGREDIENTS

- pepper
- salt
- ¾ tsp. paprika
- 1½ tbsps. mustard
- 2¼ tbsps. mayo
- 6 chopped bacon slices
- 9 hard-boiled eggs

STEP 1

Take out a skillet and heat it up to cook the bacon until crisp. Move to a plate with some paper towels to drain.

STEP 2

Halve the eggs and scoop out the yolks. Arrange the halves on a plater. Mash the yolks with paprika, mayo, salt, pepper, and mustard.

STEP 3

Dice the bacon, and then add some into the yolk mixture to stir well.

STEP 4

Spoon the yolk back into the egg whites and divide the rest of the bacon among them. Serve or store.

NUTRITIONAL INFORMATION

283 Calories, 21g Fats, 3g Net Carbs, and 20g Protein

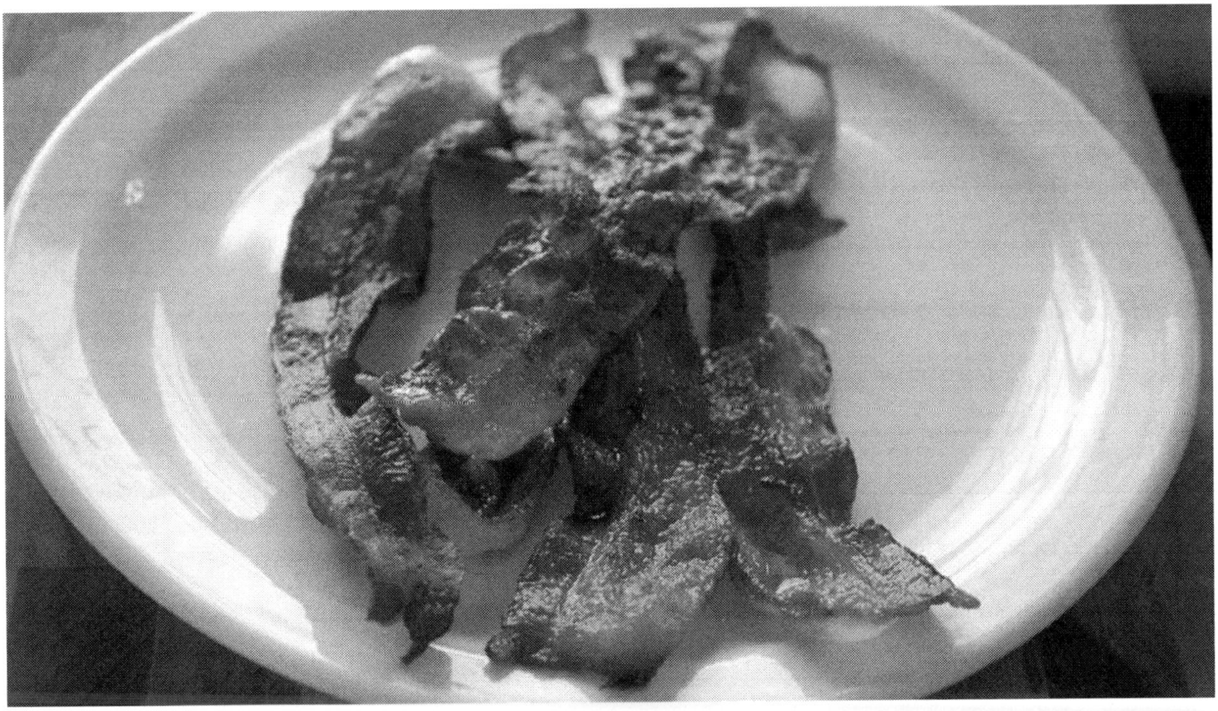

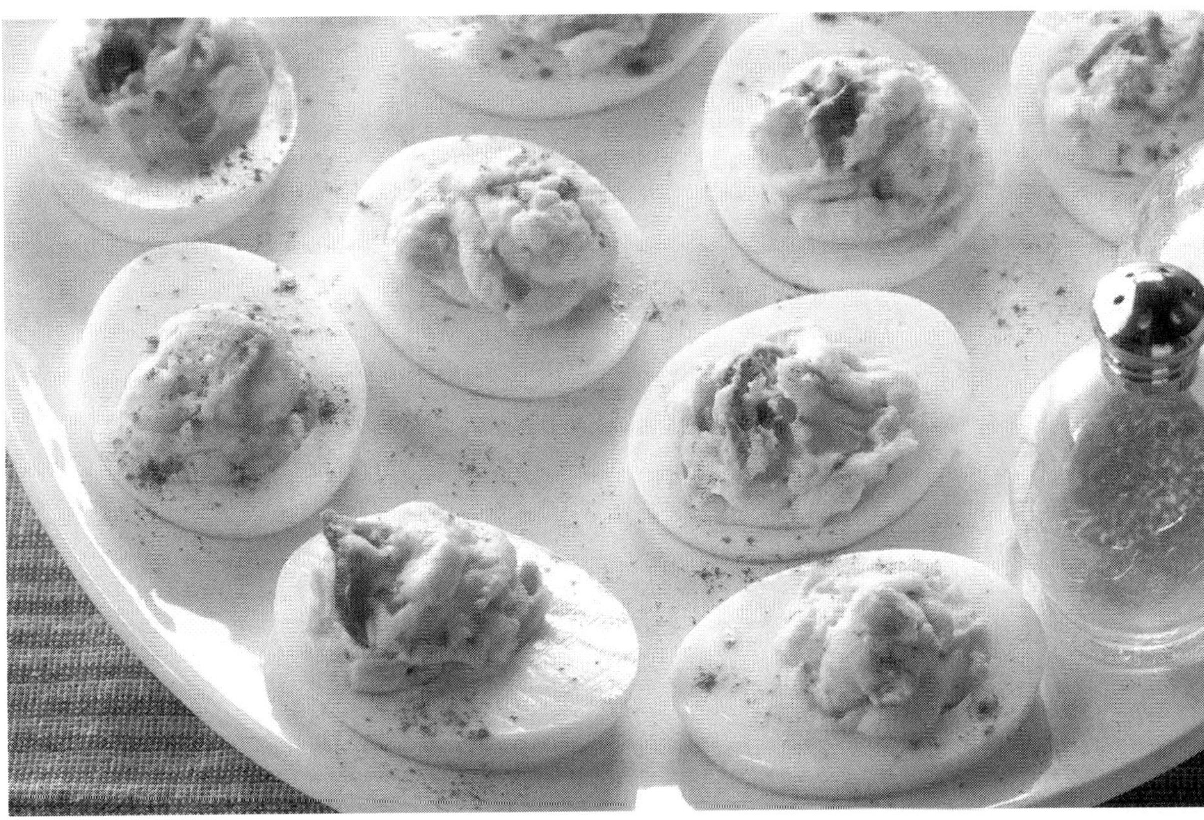

NOODLES CARBONARA

Cooking Difficulty: 3/10	Cooking Time: 21 minutes	Servings: 4

INGREDIENTS

- 3 packets shirataki noodles
- 5 oz. chopped bacon
- 1½ tbsps. butter
- 2 garlic cloves
- 1 c. grated cheese
- 3 eggs

STEP 1

Melt the butter in a pan and then add the bacon and cook until crispy. Then add in the noodles and the garlic.

STEP 2

Stir the noodles as they are heating up. While those are cooking, bring out a new bowl and beat the eggs with some of the cheese.

STEP 3

Add the cooked noodles to a new bowl. Stir the egg and cheese mixture into this, watching for the sauce to thicken.

STEP 4

Top with the parsley and the rest of the cheese and enjoy.

NUTRITIONAL INFORMATION

361 Calories, 29g Fats, 4.5g Net Carbs, 16g Protein

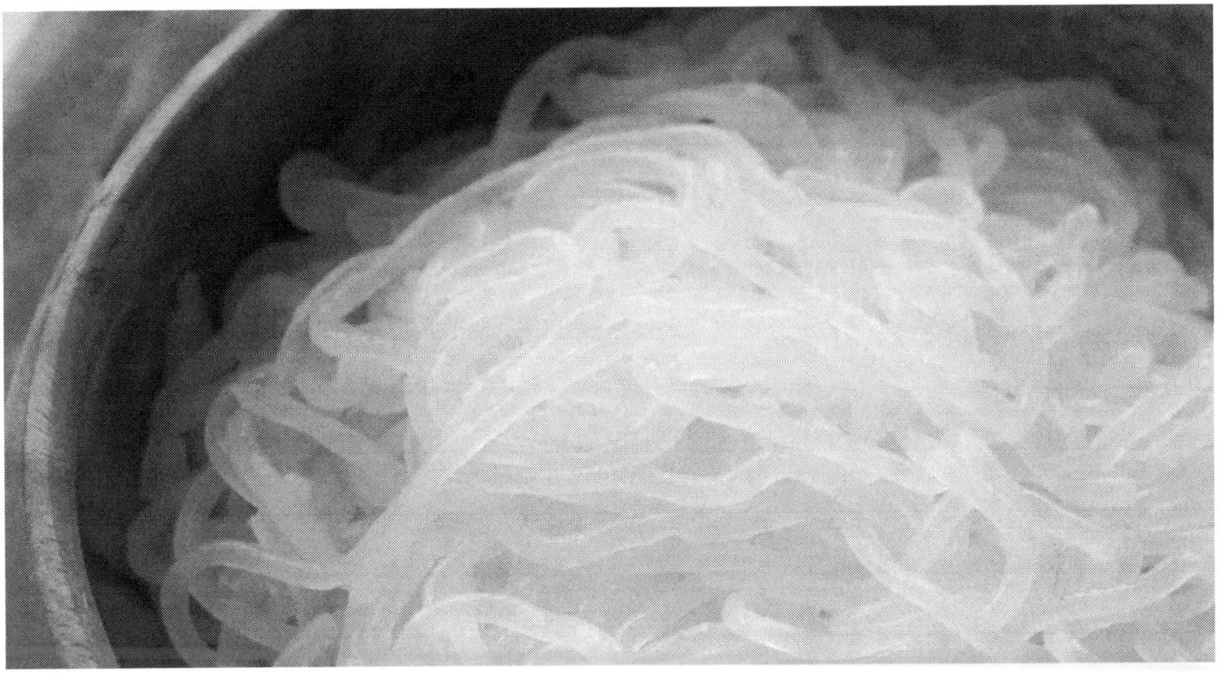

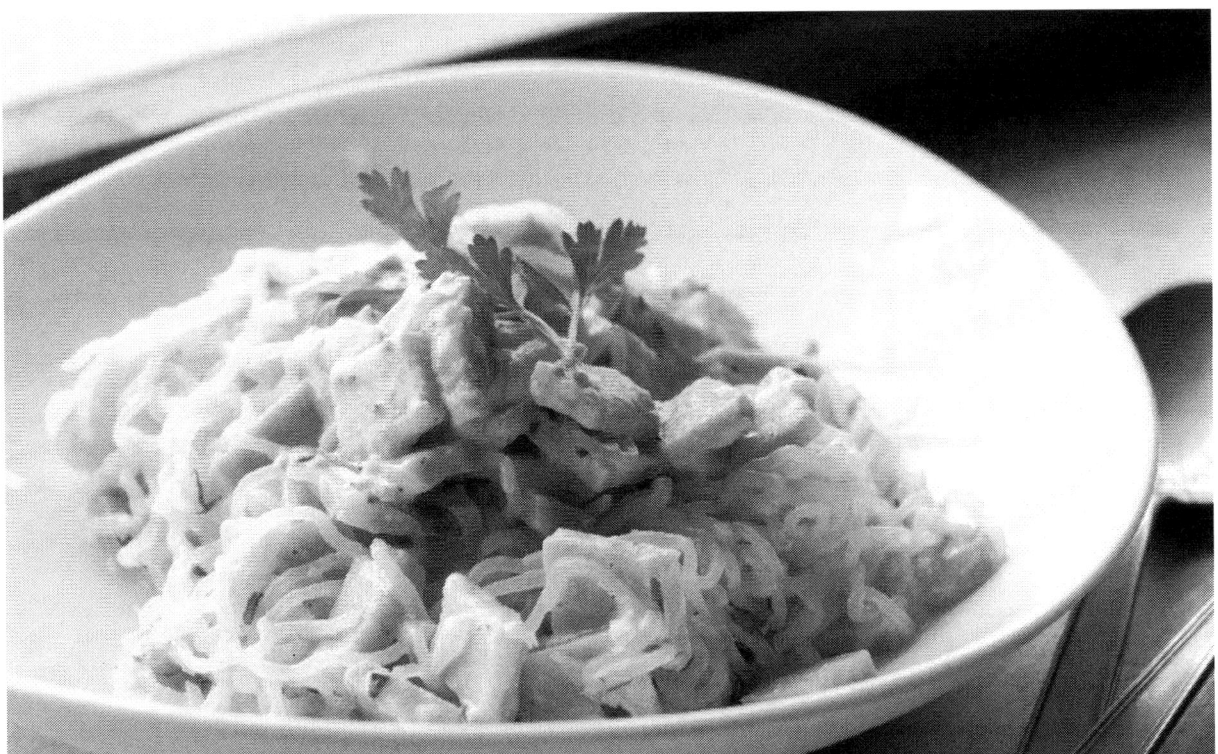

BACON BURGERS

Cooking Difficulty: 3/10	Cooking Time: 71 minutes	Servings: 12

INGREDIENTS

- pepper
- salt
- 1 tsp. onion powder
- 1 tsp. cumin powder
- 12 raw sausage patties
- 1-inch cubes of cheddar cheese
- 12 bacon

STEP 1

Allow the oven to heat up to 350 degrees. Line a baking tray with some parchment paper. Add the sausage patties to this tray.

STEP 2

Add the seasonings to the sausage, and then place a piece of the cheese in the middle of the patties. Wrap the sausage around the cheese into a ball. Wrap the sausage patties in bacon.

STEP 3

Add the baking pan into the oven. After an hour, take them out and let them cool down.

NUTRITIONAL INFORMATION

250 Calories, 20g Fats, 1g Net Carbs, and 14g Protein

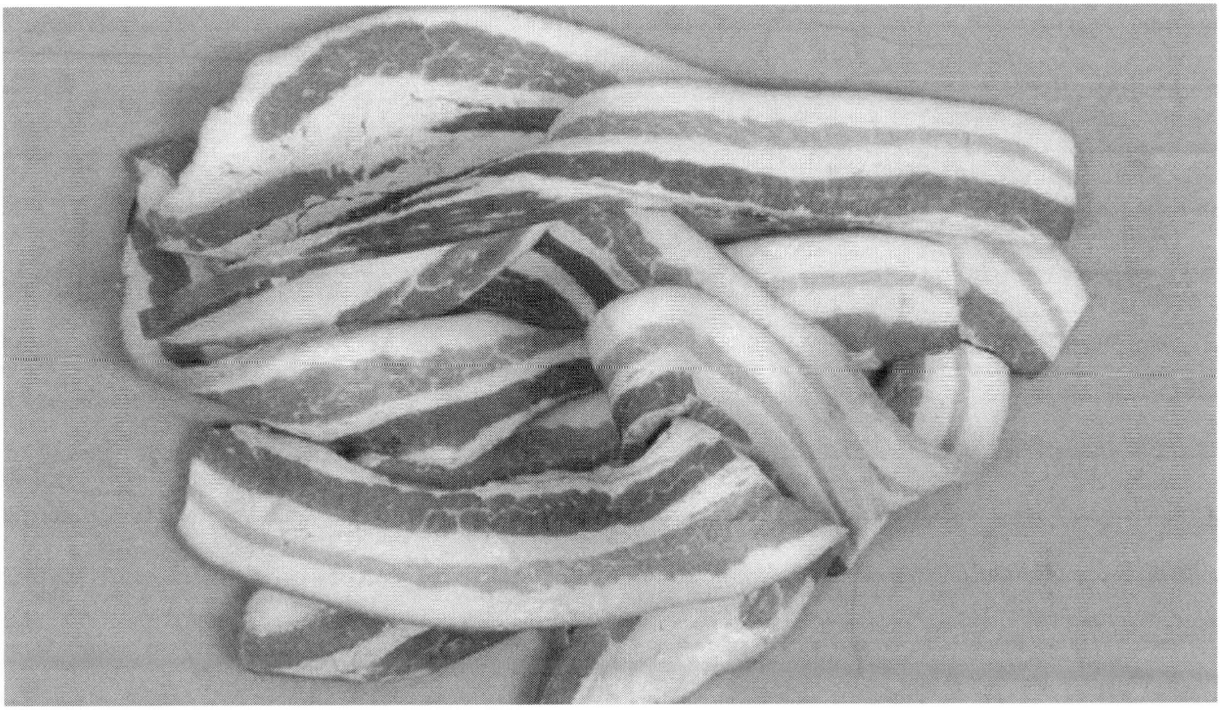
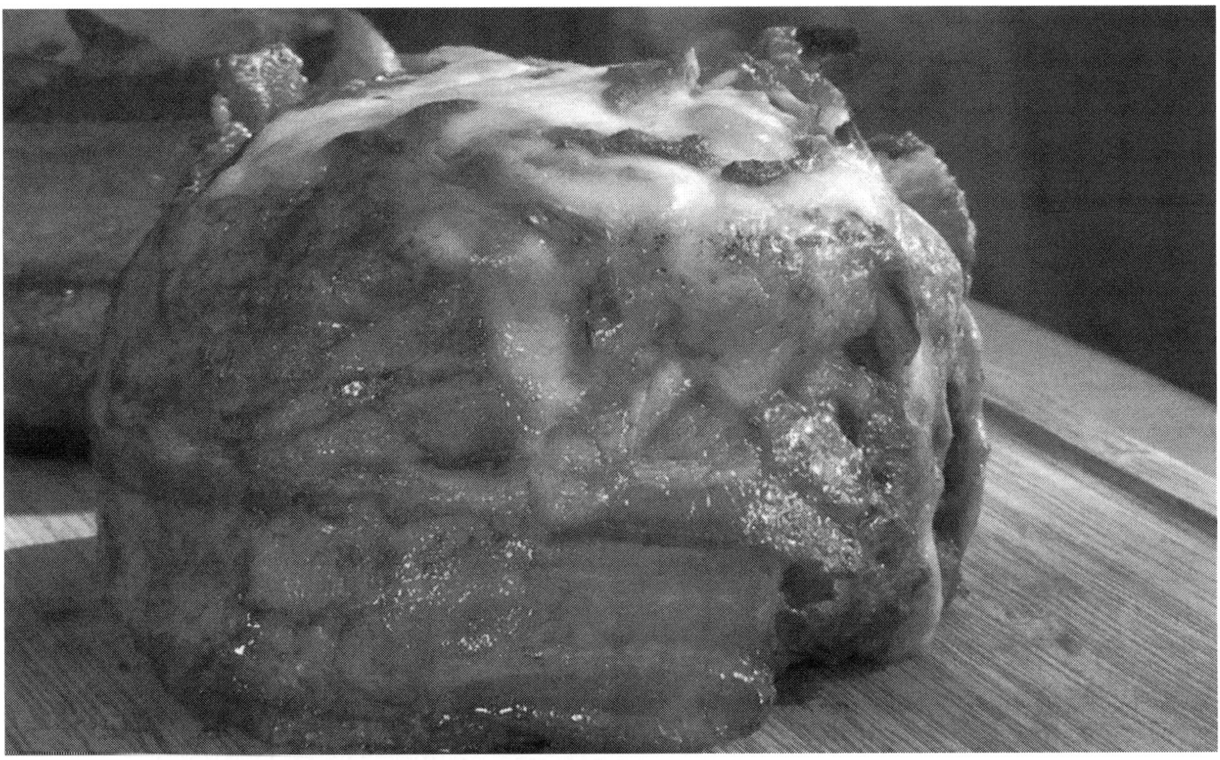

CHICKEN AND SPROUT BAKE

Cooking Difficulty: 3/10	Cooking Time: 244 minutes	Servings: 6

INGREDIENTS

- 500g brussels sprouts
- 6 chicken legs or thighs
- 500g mushrooms
- 1 diced onion
- 1½ c. milk
- 1 c. cream
- salt
- pepper

STEP 1

Mix the milk, cream, and seasoning.

STEP 2

Put all ingredients in an oven tray.

STEP 3

Cook at 130C for 4h.

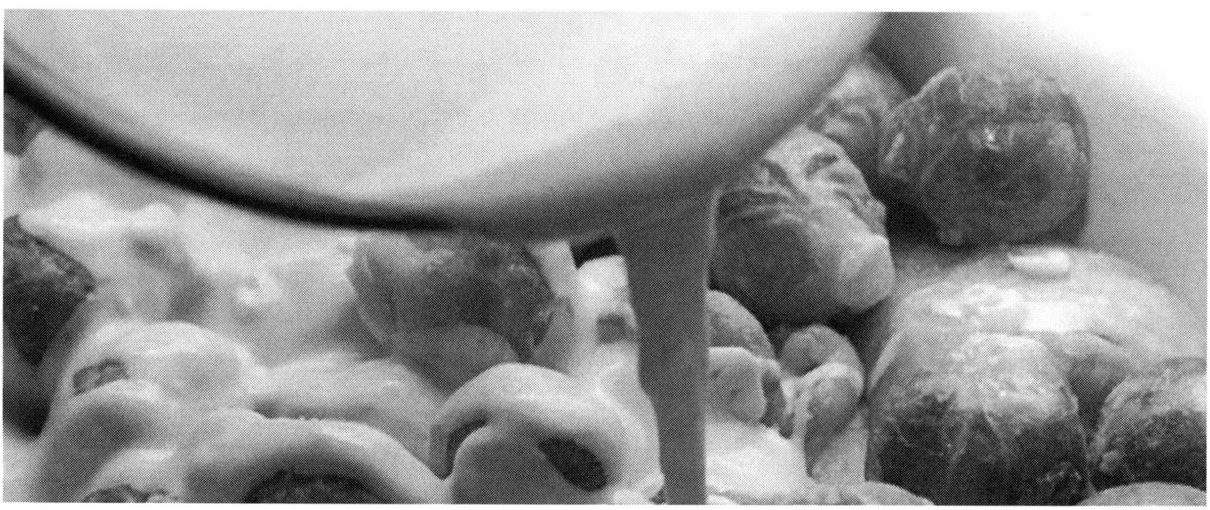

NUTRITIONAL INFORMATION

450 Calories, 30g Fats, 2g Net Carbs, 35g Protein

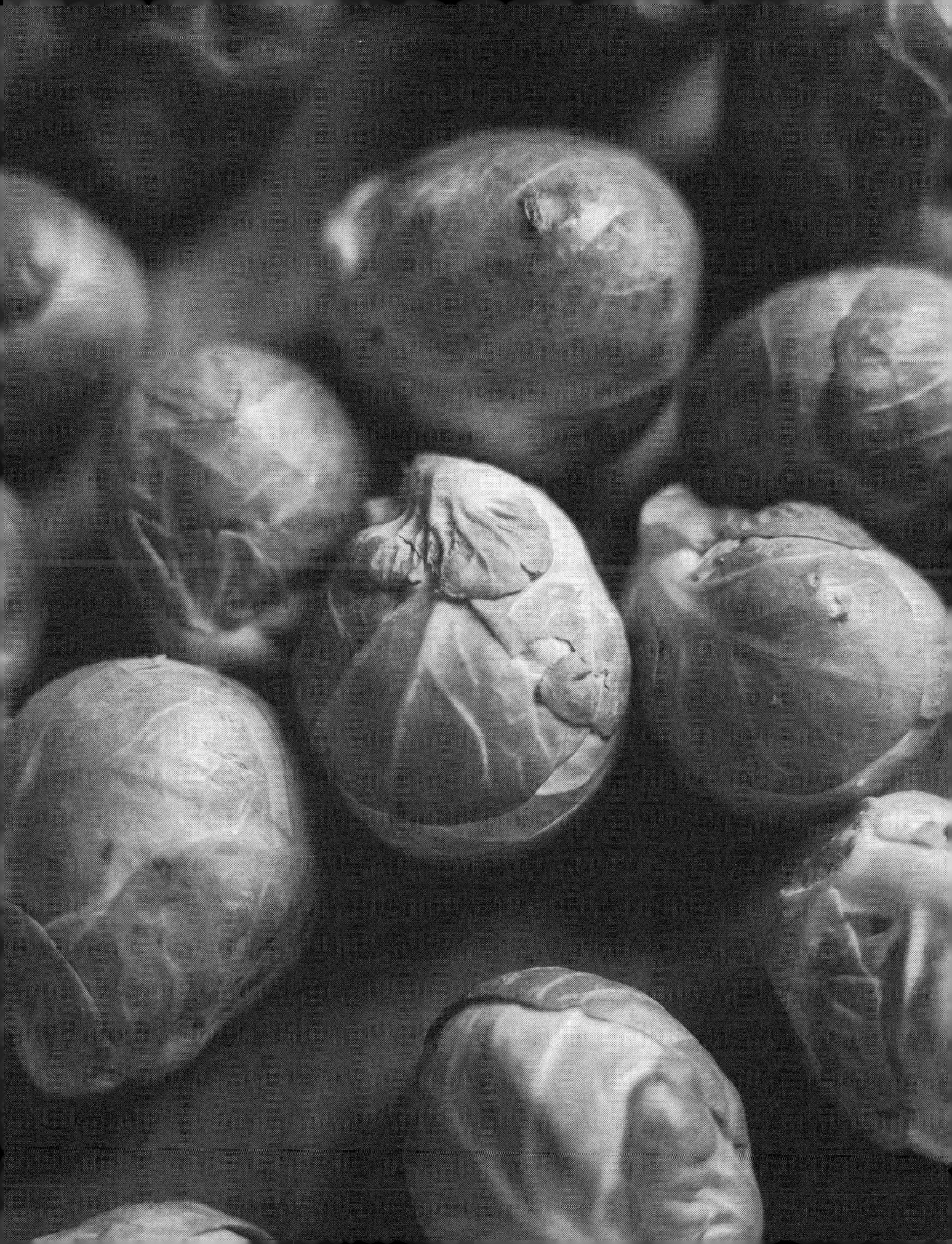

SHRIMP TUSCANY

Cooking Difficulty: 2/10	Cooking Time: 15 minutes	Servings: 4

INGREDIENTS

- ¼ c. baby kale
- 5 sun-dried tomatoes
- ½ c. parmesan
- 1 tsp. salt
- 1 tsp. dried basil
- 2 crushed garlic cloves
- ½ c. whole milk
- 1 c. cued cream cheese
- 1 tsp. butter
- 1 lb. raw shrimp

STEP 1

Melt up the butter in a pan and add in the shrimp. Cook for 30 seconds and then turn them around. Cook until they turn pink.

STEP 2

Add in the cream cheese and milk into the pan and increase the heat. Stir, so the cheese melts completely.

STEP 3

Add in the basil, salt, and garlic and keep cooking. Allow the dish to simmer so that the sauce can thicken.

STEP 4

Add in the tomatoes and kale and then serve.

NUTRITIONAL INFORMATION

298 Calories, 18g Fats, 6.5g Net Carbs, 23g Protein

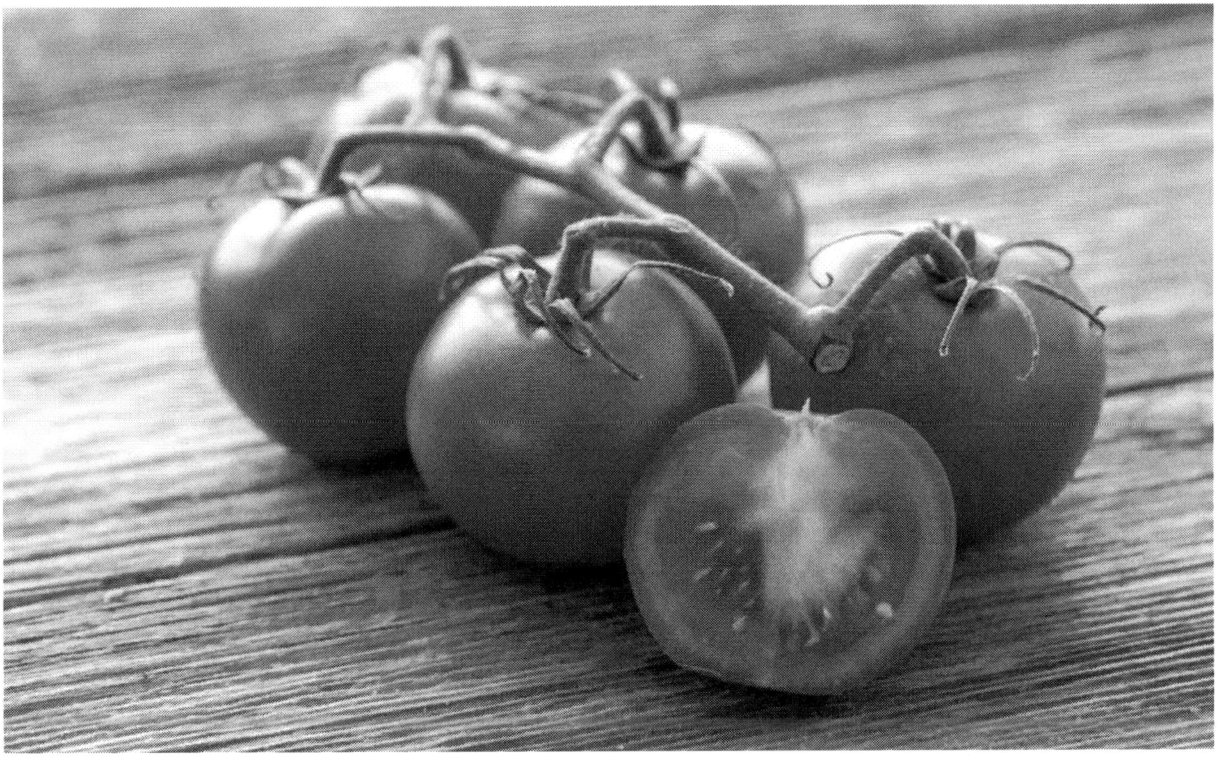

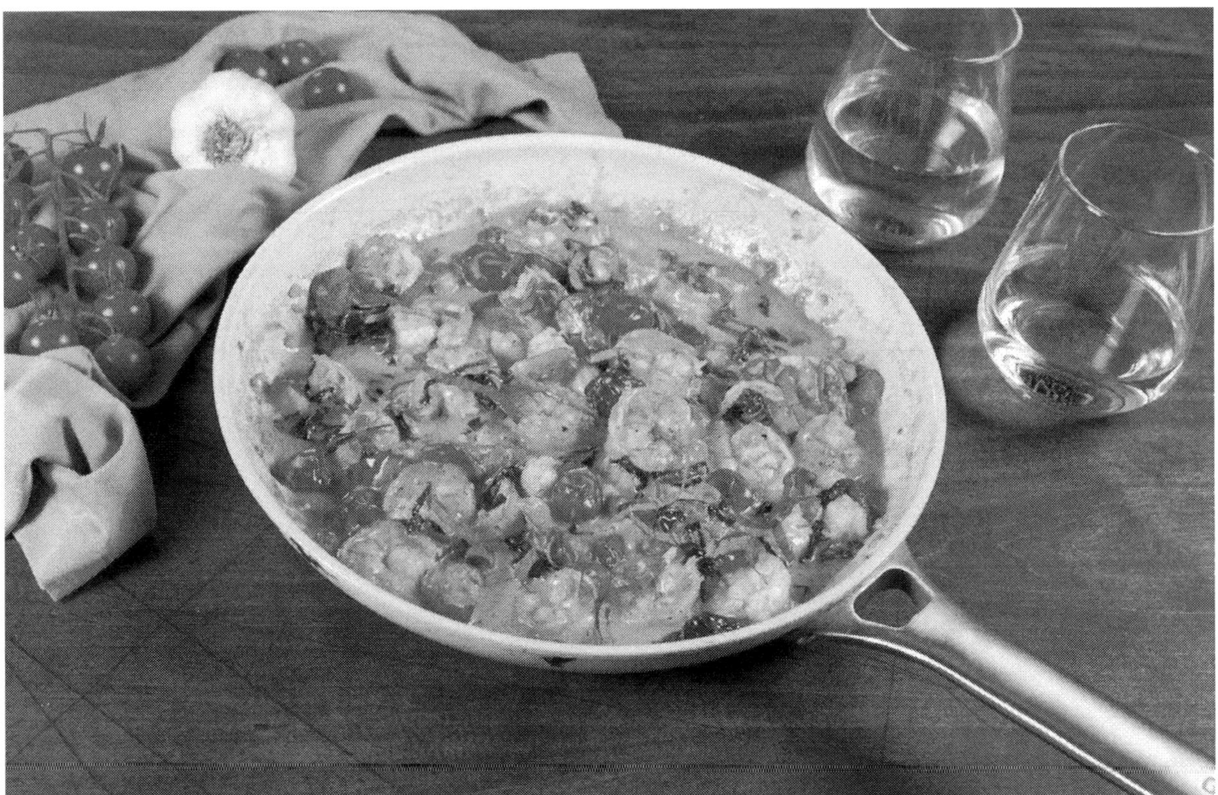

GARLIC PORK CHOPS

Cooking Difficulty: 4/10	Cooking Time: 23 minutes	Servings: 4

INGREDIENTS

- 1 chopped onion
- 1 tsp. crushed garlic
- 1 tbsp. paprika
- 4 pork chops
- 1 tbsp. chopped parsley
- ½ c. heavy cream
- 1 tbsp. butter
- 1 c. sliced mushrooms
- 2 tbsps. coconut oil
- ¼ tsp. cayenne pepper
- 1 tsp. salt
- 1 tsp. pepper

STEP 1

Mix together the seasonings with a third of the onion. Sprinkle on both chops and rub it in.

STEP 2

Heat up some coconut oil and brown the chops for a few minutes on both sides. Set them to the side.

STEP 3

Add in the rest of the mushrooms and onions and cook another four minutes to make the onions clear.

STEP 4

In a new pan, whisk the butter and cream on low heat. Place the chops into the cream sauce and cook for another five minutes. Add mushrooms and serve.

NUTRITIONAL INFORMATION

481 Calories, 32g Fats, 4g Net Carbs, 15g Protein

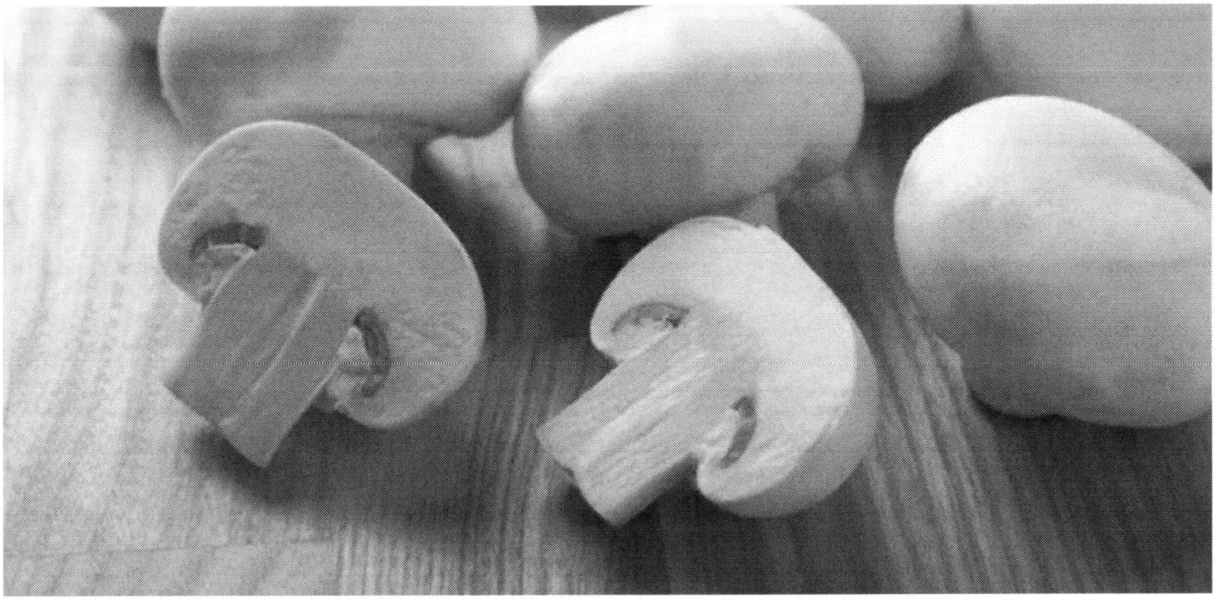

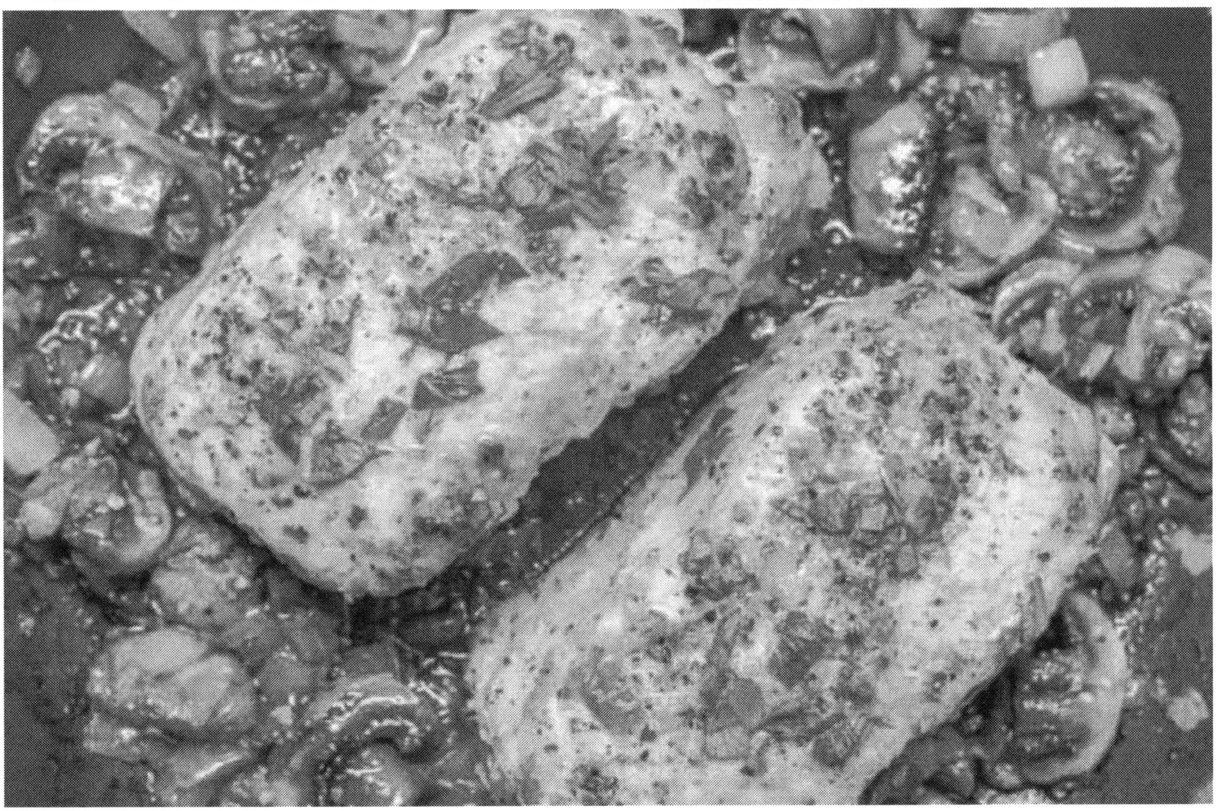

ITALIAN MEATBALLS

Cooking Difficulty: 4/10	Cooking Time: 34 minutes	Servings: 4

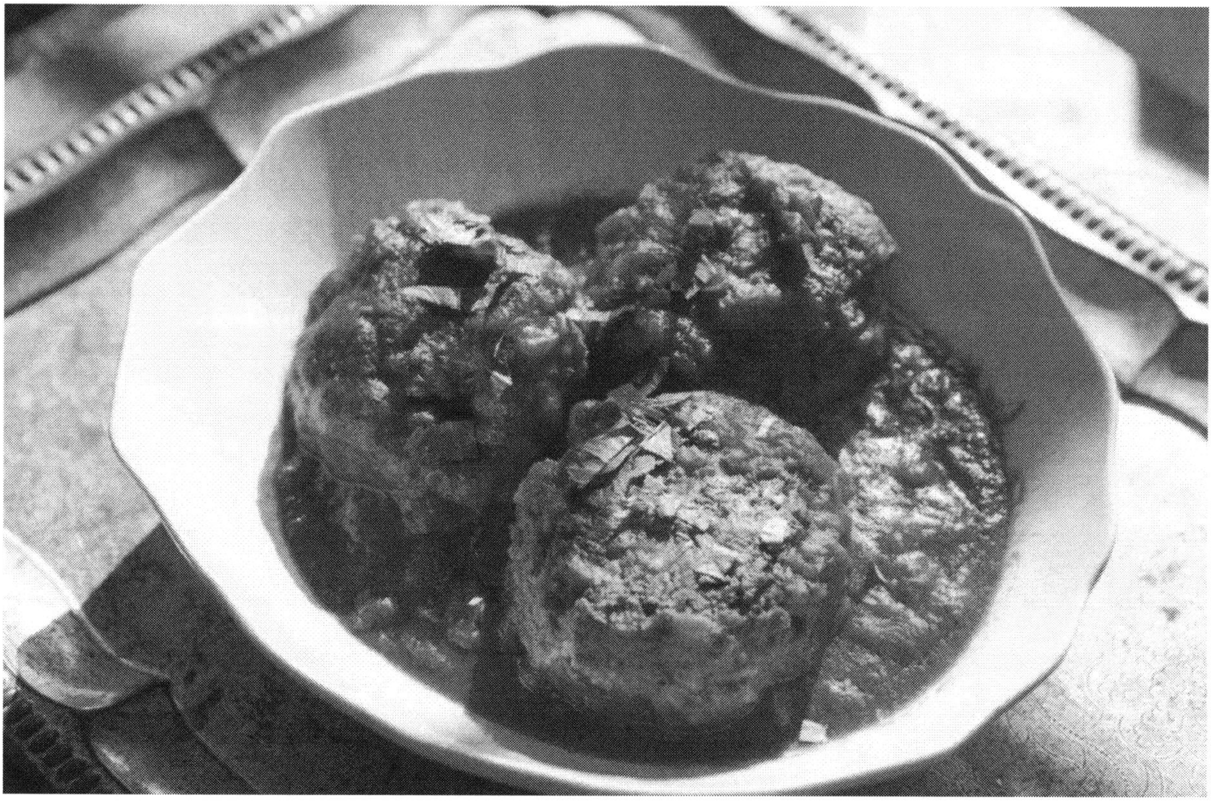

NUTRITIONAL INFORMATION

380 Calories, 23g Fats, 8g Net Carbs, 25g Protein

INGREDIENTS

- 1 tsp. dried thyme
- 1 tsp. dried oregano
- ½ c. sliced mozzarella
- 1 can peeled tomatoes
- 1 lb. minced beef
- 1 handful basil
- 1 tbsp. tomato paste
- 2 crushed garlic cloves
- ½ c. diced red onion, diced

STEP 1

Allow the oven to heat up to 350 degrees. Take out a bowl and mix together the ground beef and herbs. Form into 16 meatballs.

STEP 2

Fry these in a skillet for five minutes to make them brown. Take a bit of the cooking juices and set to the side.

STEP 3

Add the garlic, tomato paste, onion, and tinned tomatoes into the ban. Simmer this for another ten minutes.

STEP 4

Place the meatballs into a dish and top with this sauce. Break up the cheese and spread it on the tomato sauce.

STEP 5

Cover the dish with some foil and place in the oven. Bake for 20 minutes. Take the foil off and bake a bit longer.

STEP 6

Serve with a salad.

SAVORY BUTTERNUT SQUASH SOUP

Cooking Difficulty: 3/10	Cooking Time: 26 minutes	Servings: 4

INGREDIENTS

- ½ lb. cubed butternut squash
- 1 bay leaf
- 2 minced garlic cloves
- 2 c. organic chicken broth
- ¼ c. heavy cream
- 2½ tbsps. olive oil
- ½ tsp. sea salt

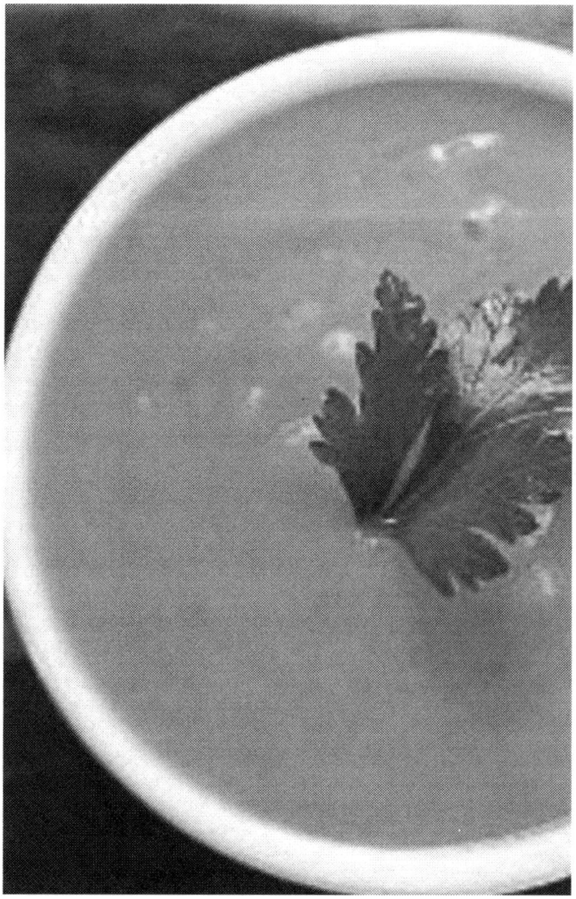

NUTRITIONAL INFORMATION

179 Calories, 14g Fats, 6g Net Carbs, 8g Protein.

STEP 1

Place a saucepan over medium flame and heat through. Once hot, add ½ tablespoon of olive oil and swirl to coat.

STEP 2

Stir the butternut squash and garlic into the saucepan and sauté for about 5 minutes or until the garlic is lightly toasted.

STEP 3

Pour the chicken broth into the saucepan along with the remaining olive oil. Add the bay leaf, then bring to a boil. Once boiling, reduce to a simmer.

STEP 4

Simmer the mixture for about 20 minutes or until the butternut squash is completely tender.

STEP 5

Take out and discard the bay leaf, then turn off the heat and allow to cool slightly. Once cooled, blend using an immersion blender or high power blender until smooth.

STEP 6

Pour in the cream and blend again until smooth. Then, return to the saucepan and reheat over the medium-low flame.

STEP 7

Season the soup to taste with salt then divide into individual servings. Allow cooling slightly, then seal tightly. Refrigerate for up to 3 days. Reheat before serving.

KETO CAESAR SALAD

Cooking Difficulty:	Cooking Time:	Servings:
2/10	13 minutes	6

INGREDIENTS

- 12 c. chopped romaine lettuce
- 1/3 c. extra virgin olive oil
- 1/3 c. grated parmesan cheese
- 3 tbsps. squeezed lemon juice
- 1½ tbsps. mayonnaise
- 1/3 tsp. anchovy paste
- 1/3 tsp. garlic powder
- black pepper

STEP 1

Combine the lemon juice, olive oil, anchovy paste, garlic powder, and mayonnaise in an airtight container. Whisk well until thoroughly combined. Divide into 6 equal servings in small airtight containers and refrigerate for up to 3 days.

STEP 2

In a large bowl, toss together the lettuce and Parmesan cheese. Season lightly with black pepper and toss again to coat. Divide into 6 airtight containers, then cover and refrigerate for up to 3 days.

STEP 3

Right before serving, add the dressing to the salad. Toss to coat, then serve right away.

NUTRITIONAL INFORMATION

93 Calories, 7g Fats, 6g Net Carbs, and 3g Protein

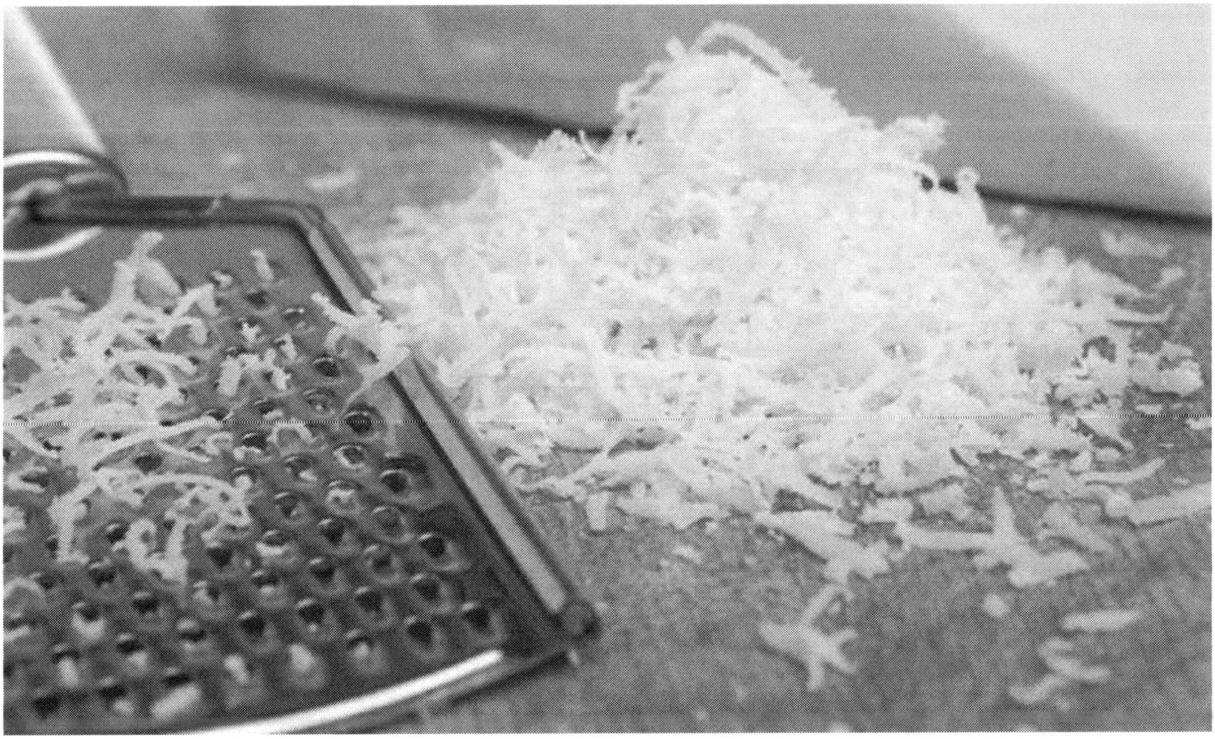

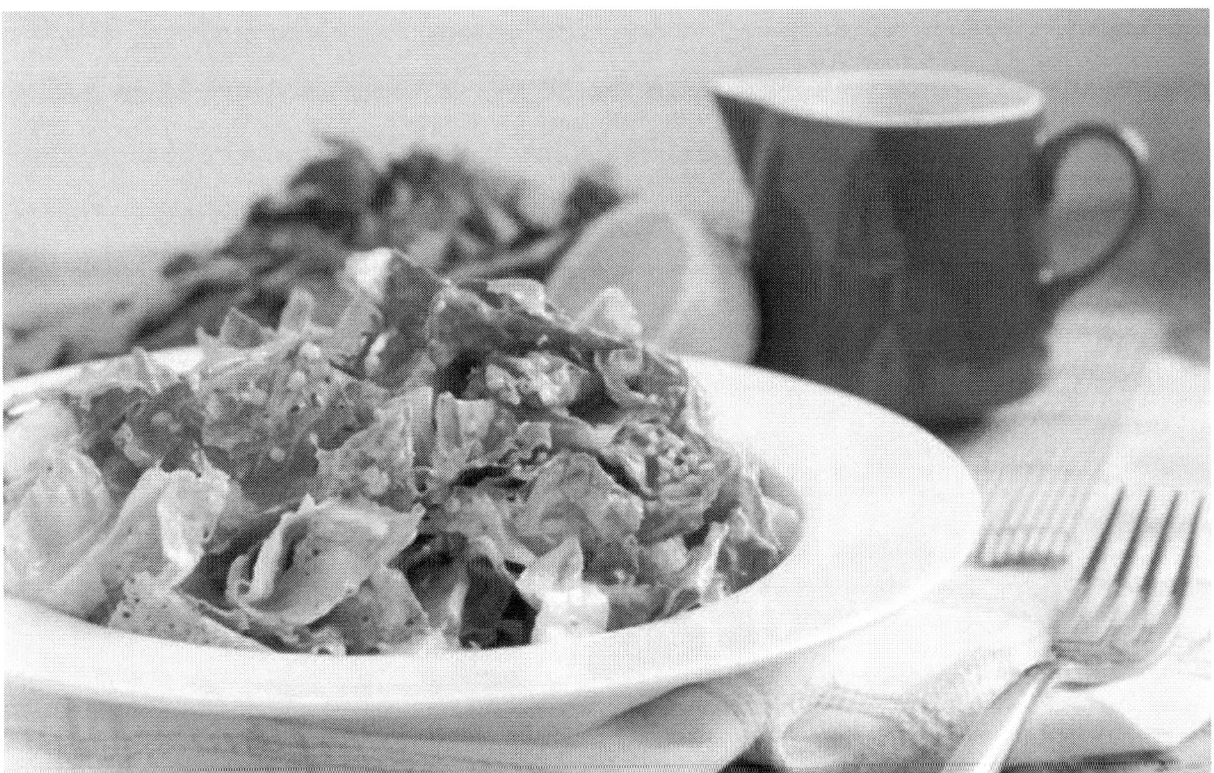

BEEF WELLY

Cooking Difficulty: 3/10	Cooking Time: 27 minutes	Servings: 2

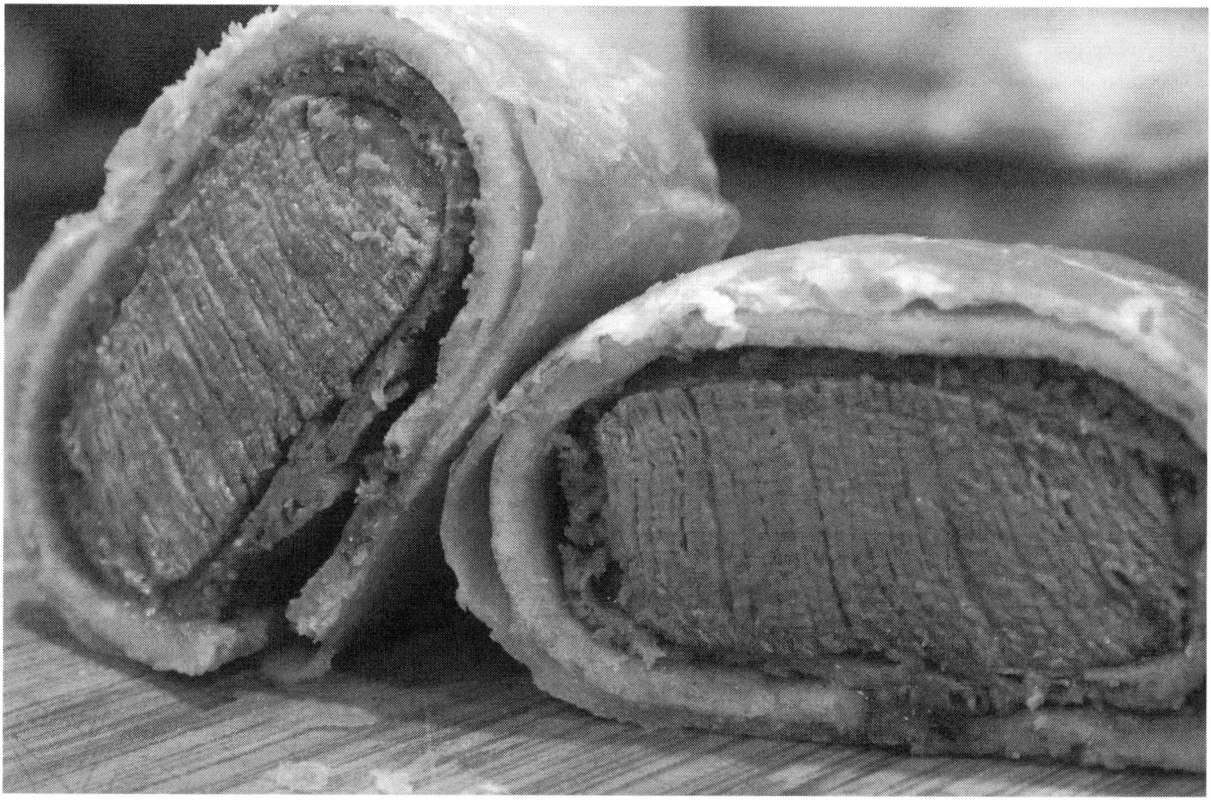

NUTRITIONAL INFORMATION

307 Calories, 22g Fats, 2.5g Net Carbs, 26g Protein

INGREDIENTS

- ½ c. almond flour
- 1 c. mozzarella cheese
- 4 tbsps. liver pate
- 1 tbsp. butter
- 2 tenderloin steaks

STEP 1

Season the steaks. Melt some butter in a pan and let it heat up before adding the steaks to the pan. Sear it on all sides and then let them cool down.

STEP 2

Heat up some mozzarella in the microwave for a minute. Add in the almond flour to form a dough.

STEP 3

Place this dough between two pieces of parchment paper and then roll it flat. Place some pate on the dough and spread it out.

STEP 4

Cut the dough so that it can make a ball around the meat. Add some meat into the dough and cut it, wrapping it around the meat. Do this with the other piece of meat as well.

STEP 5

Allow the oven to heat up to 400 degrees. Place into the oven and let it bake. After 20 minutes, it is done.

MEXICAN CASSEROLE

Cooking Difficulty: 4/10	Cooking Time: 45 minutes	Servings: 12

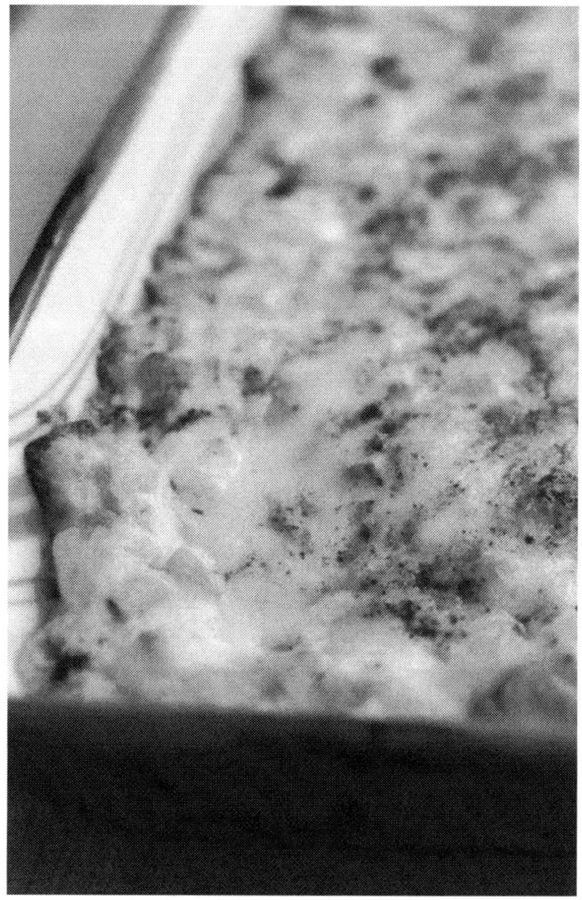

INGREDIENTS

- ½ tsp. cumin
- 1 head cauliflower
- ½ white onion
- ½ tsp. chili powder
- 1 green bell pepper
- 1½ c. parmesan
- 1 hashed bell pepper
- 4 chopped cherry tomatoes

NUTRITIONAL INFORMATION

69 Calories, 30g Total Fats, 4.5g Carbs, 3.56g Protein

STEP 1

Ensure your oven is set to 350 degrees Fahrenheit.

STEP 2

Place the skillet on top of the stove over a burner set to medium heat.

STEP 3

Roast the chili powder, pepper, cumin, and onion, stirring regularly until the veggies are fully cooked.

STEP 4

Dice the cauliflower. Cook it in the microwave for 3 minutes.

STEP 5

Put the tomatoes and 1 cup of the cheese in with the cauliflower. Mix.

STEP 6

Mix the results with the vegetables.

STEP 7

Using cooking spray, coat a baking dish.

STEP 8

Add the vegetable mixture to the baking dish.

STEP 9

Add the rest of the cheese.

STEP 10

Place the dish in the oven and let it cook for approximately 40 minutes.

STEP 11

Garnish as dcsircd.

BASIL TOMATO SALMON

Cooking Difficulty: 2/10	Cooking Time: 23 minutes	Servings: 2

INGREDIENTS

- 2 boneless salmon fillets
- tbsps. olive oil
- 1 thinly sliced tomato
- 1 tbsp. basil, dried
- 2 tbsps. parmesan cheese, grated

STEP 1

Preheat the oven to 375F.

STEP 2

Take an aluminum foil and line the baking sheet and grease it with nonstick cooking spray.

STEP 3

Place the salmon on the foil; sprinkle with the basil; top with the tomato; drizzle with the olive oil, or sprinkle with parmesan.

STEP 4

Bake for about 20 minutes or until the salmon center is opaque, and the cheese is lightly browned on top.

NUTRITIONAL INFORMATION

374 Calories, 41.6g Fats, 1.8g Net Carbs, 37.9g Protein

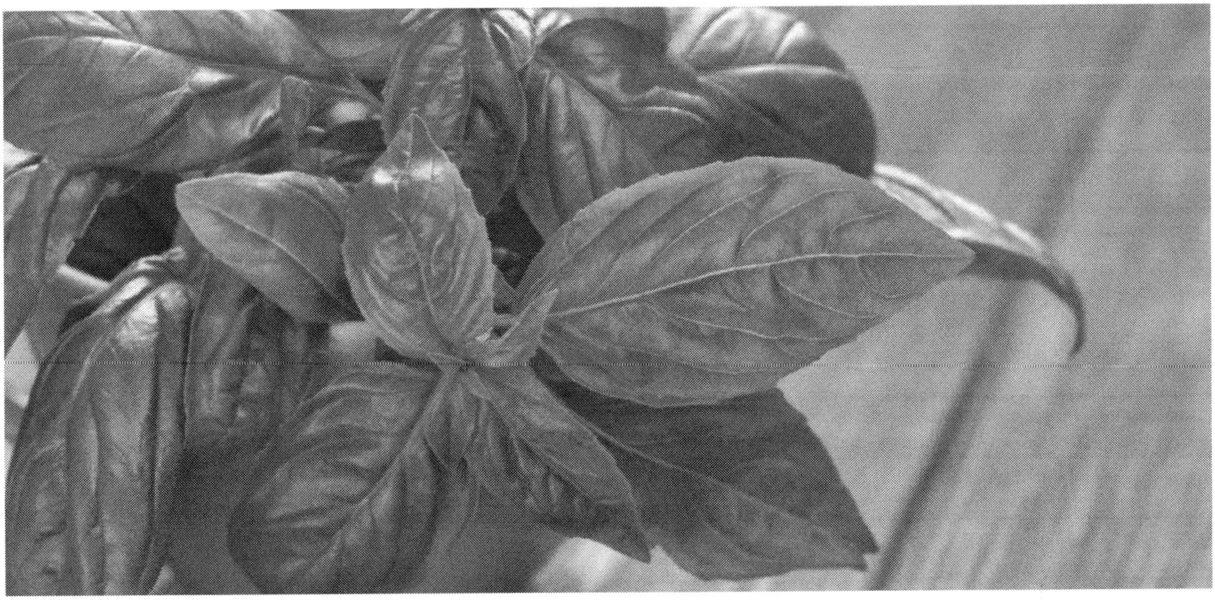

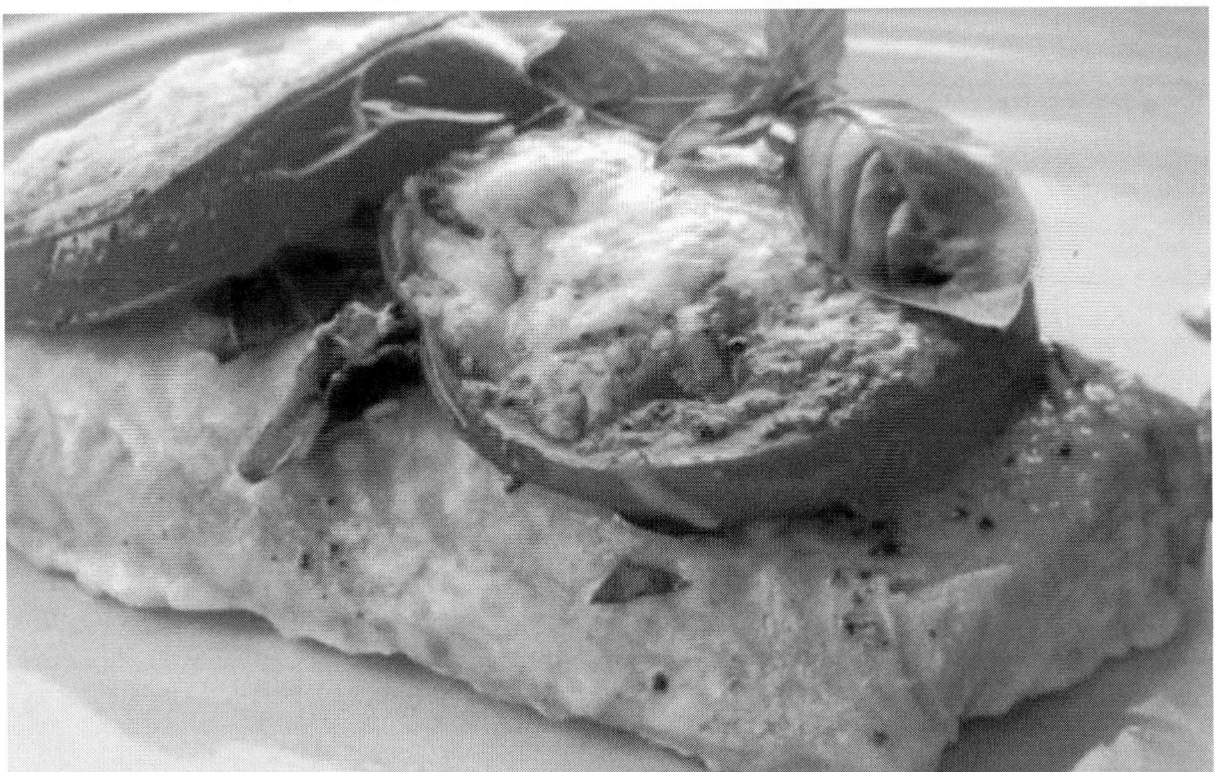

FRIED CHEESY AVOCADO WEDGES

Cooking Difficulty: 3/10	Cooking Time: 16 minutes	Servings: 4

INGREDIENTS

- 2 small eggs
- 1 large avocado
- 1/3 cup ground pork rinds
- 1/3 cup shredded parmesan cheese
- 1½ tbsps. heavy cream
- 1/3 tsp. garlic powder
- 1/3 tsp. onion powder
- 1/3 tsp. fine sea salt
- 1/3 tsp. black pepper
- sunflower oil

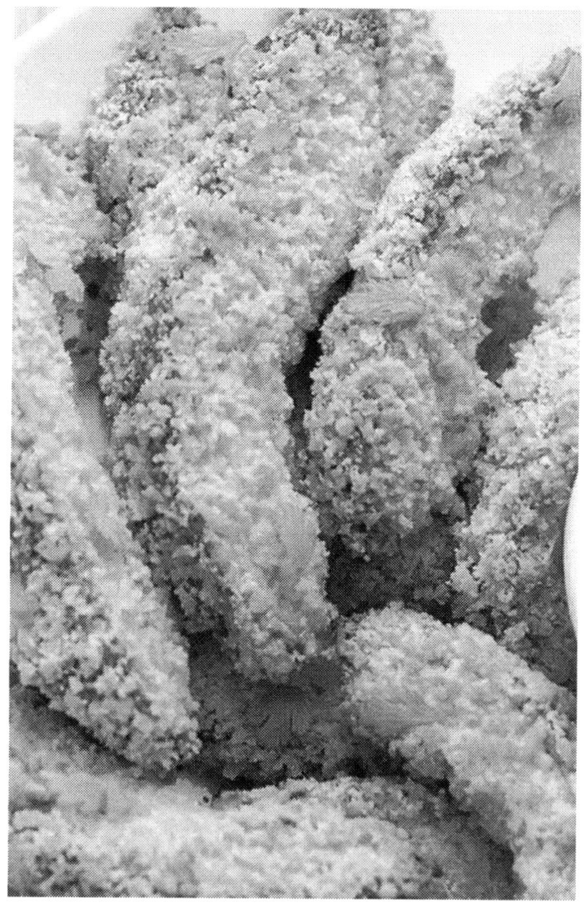

NUTRITIONAL INFORMATION

179 Calories, 14g Fats, 6g Net Carbs, 8g Protein.

STEP 1

Place a heavy-duty skillet over medium flame and add approximately 1 ½ inch of oil. Heat the oil to 375 degrees F.

STEP 2

Meanwhile, whisk the eggs in a small bowl then mix in until smooth.

STEP 3

Halve the avocado carefully, then discard the stone. Scoop out the flesh using a spoon then slice into ½ inch thick wedges.

STEP 4

Season the avocado wedges with salt and pepper then set aside.

STEP 5

On a plate, combine the pork rinds, onion and garlic powders, and Parmesan cheese. Mix well.

STEP 6

Dip the avocado wedges in the egg mixture, then drain and dredge in the pork rind and Parmesan cheese mixture until completely covered.

STEP 7

Add the coated wedges in the hot oil and cook for 1 minute per side, or until golden brown.

STEP 8

Transfer the wedges to a platter lined with paper towels and let drain. Allow to cool slightly, then transfer to an airtight container and refrigerate for up to 2 days. Reheat before serving in hot oil, if desired.

INSTANT POT RECIPES

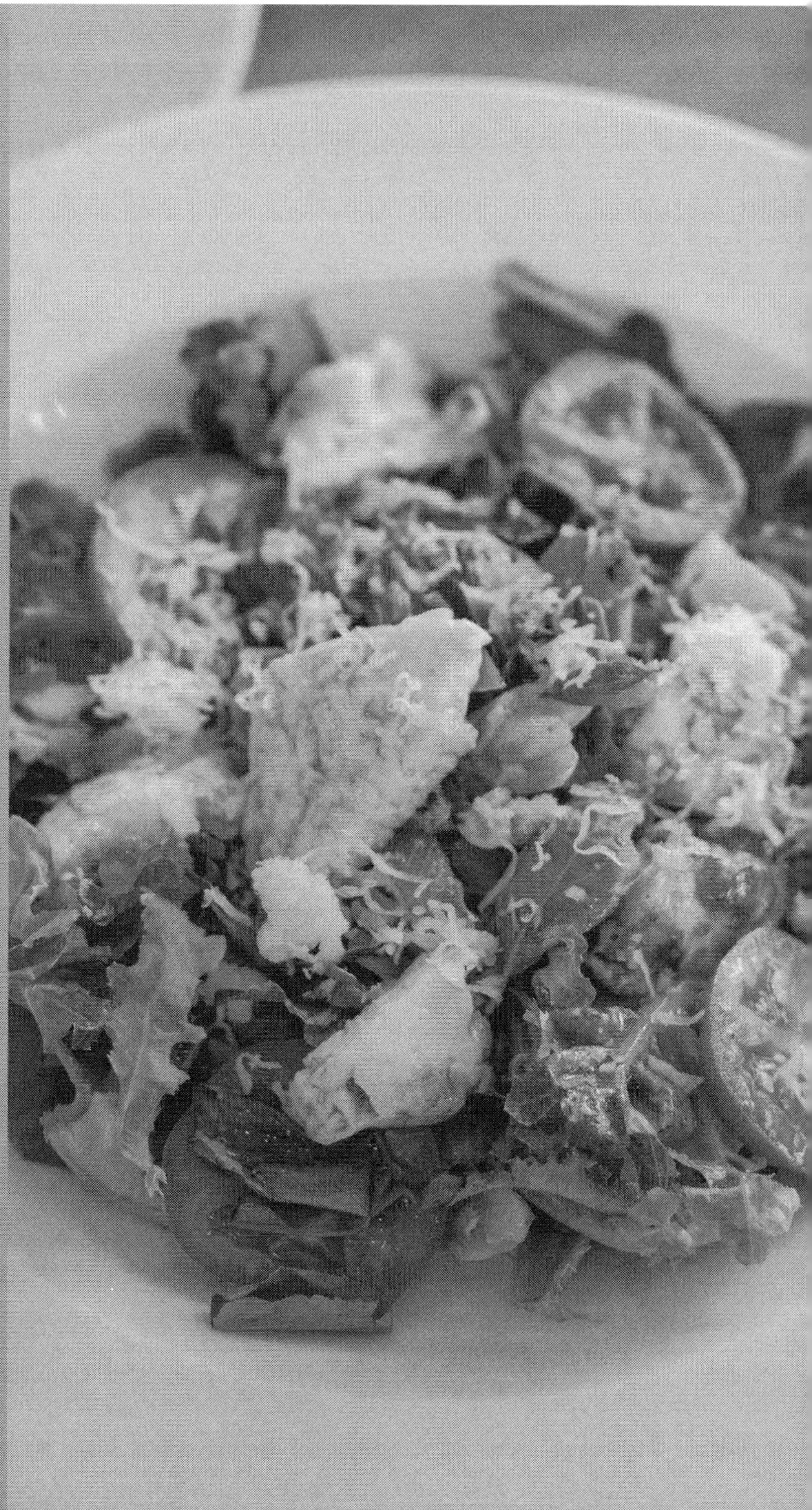

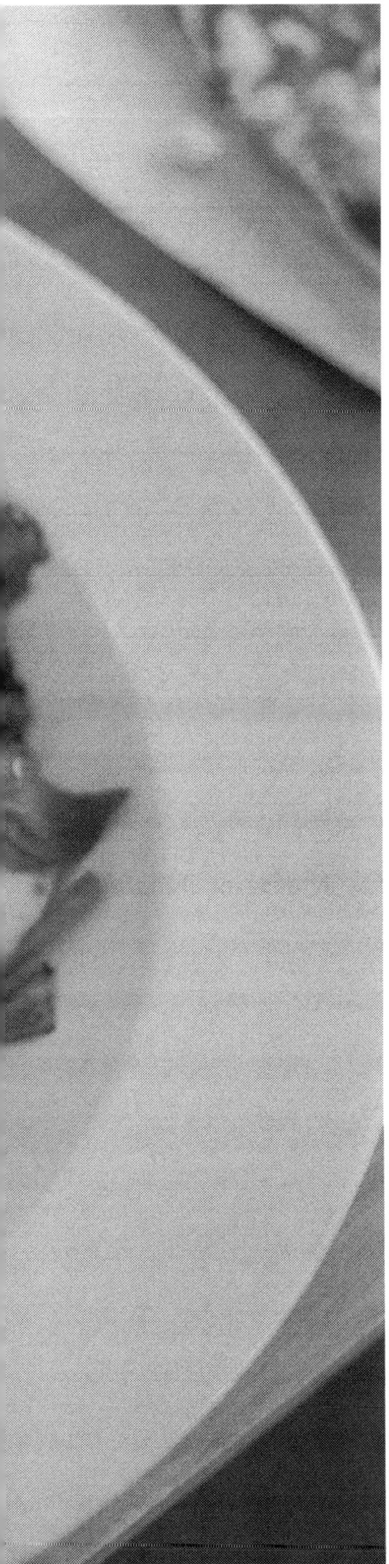

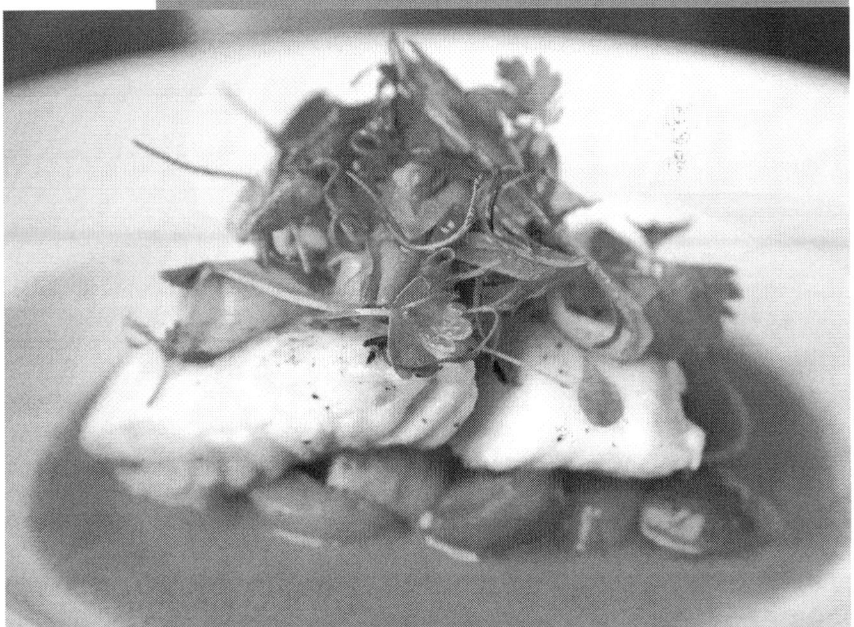

NO-CRUST TOMATO & SPINACH QUICHE

STEP 1
Pour the water into the Instant Pot.

STEP 2
Grease a baking dish with cooking spray.

STEP 3
Combine the diced tomatoes, green onions, and spinach in it.

STEP 4
Beat the eggs along with the milk, salt, and pepper.

STEP 5
Pour this mixture over the spinach and tomatoes.

STEP 6
Sprinkle with parmesan cheese and top with tomato slices.

STEP 7
Place the baking dish on the rack and close the lid.

STEP 8
Cook on HIGH for 20 minutes.

STEP 9
Wait 10 minutes before releasing the pressure quickly.

STEP 10
Serve and enjoy!

Cooking Difficulty: 3/10	Cooking Time: 32 minutes	Servings: 6

INGREDIENTS

- 1 c. diced tomatoes
- 3 c. chopped spinach
- ¼ c. grated parmesan cheese
- ½ c. milk
- 3 green onions
- 12 eggs
- ½ sliced tomato
- ½ tsp. garlic salt
- ¼ tsp. pepper

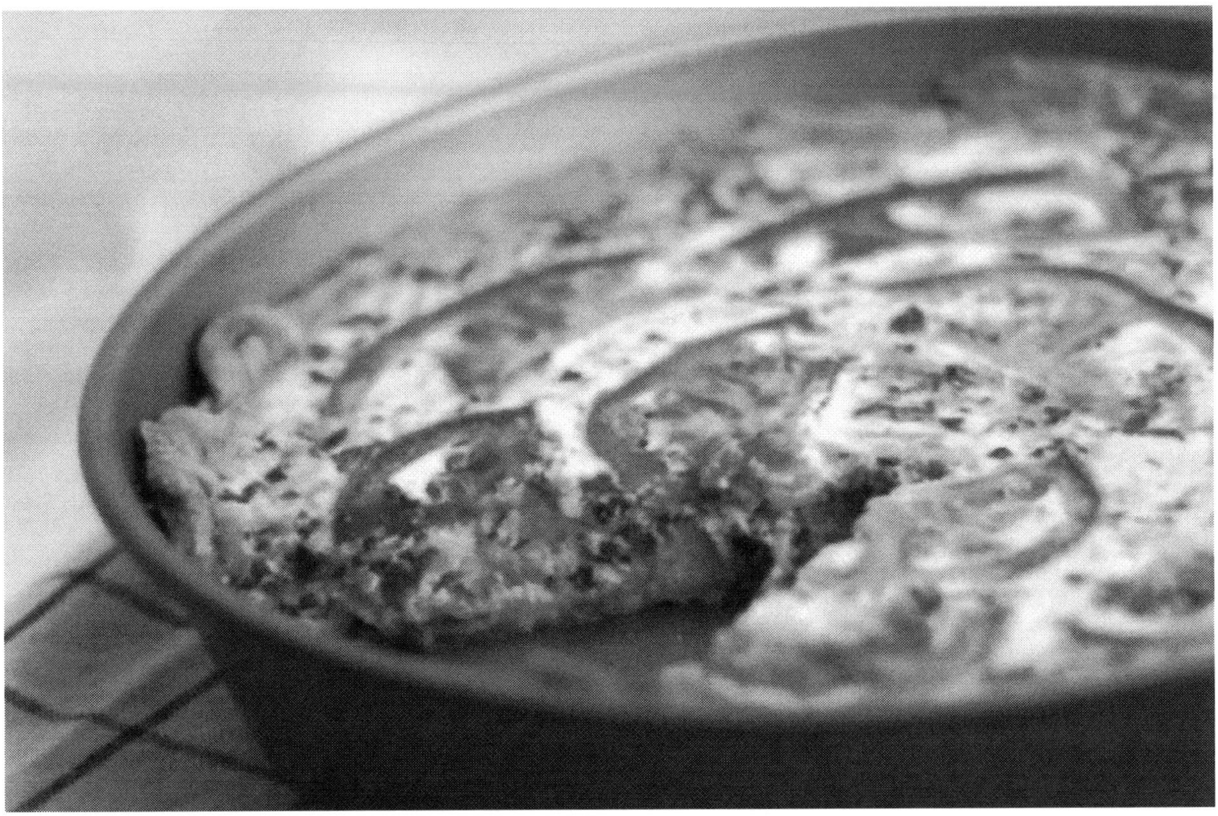

NUTRITIONAL INFORMATION

178 Calories, 11.2g Fat, 3.8g Carbs, 15.3g Protein

ALMOND AND CHIA BREAKFAST

Cooking Difficulty:	Cooking Time:	Servings:
3/10	7 minutes	2

INGREDIENTS

- 2 tbsps. chopped almonds
- 1 tbsp. chia seeds
- 2 tbsps. roasted pepitas
- 1/3 c. coconut milk
- 1/3 c. water
- a handful blueberries

STEP 1

In your food processor, mix pepitas with almonds and pulse them well.

STEP 2

In your instant pot, mix chia seeds with water and coconut milk and stir.

STEP 3

Add pepitas mix, stir, cover the pot, and cook on High for 5 minutes.

STEP 4

Add blueberries, toss a bit, divide into 2 bowls and serve for breakfast.

STEP 5

Enjoy!

NUTRITIONAL INFORMATION

183 Calories, 5g Carbs, 7g Protein, 4g Fat

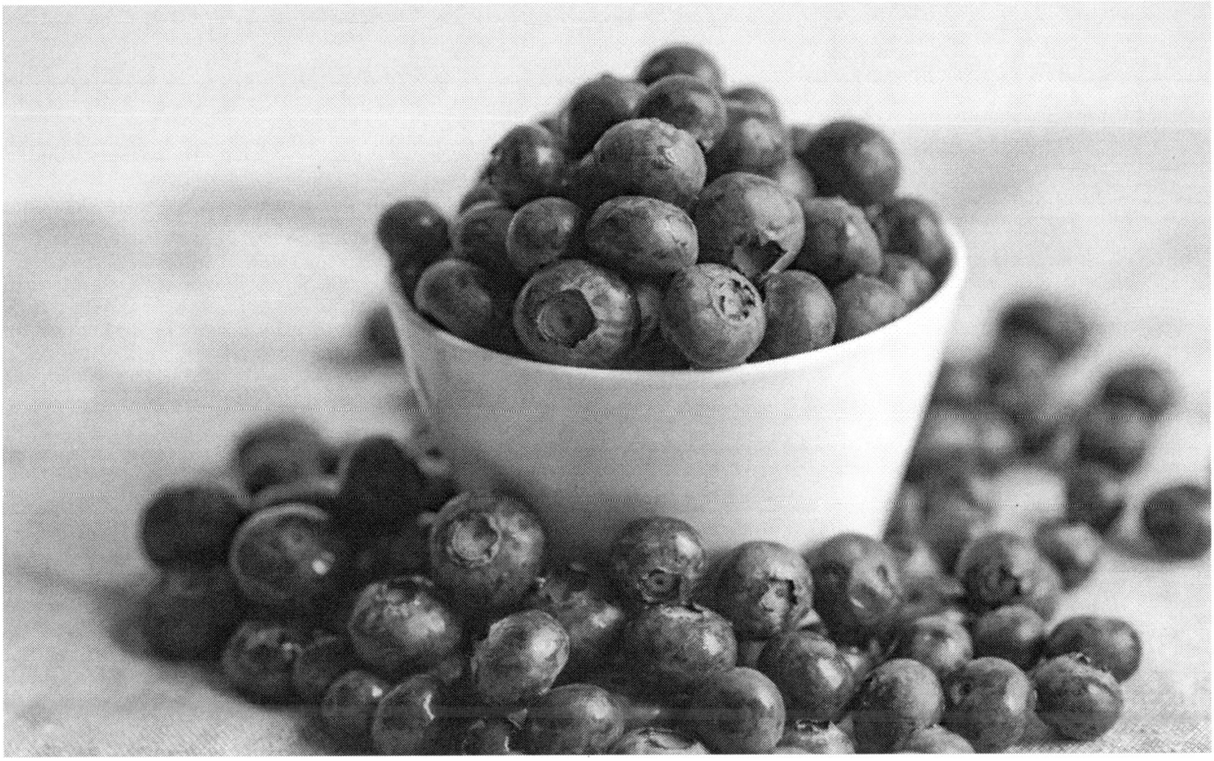

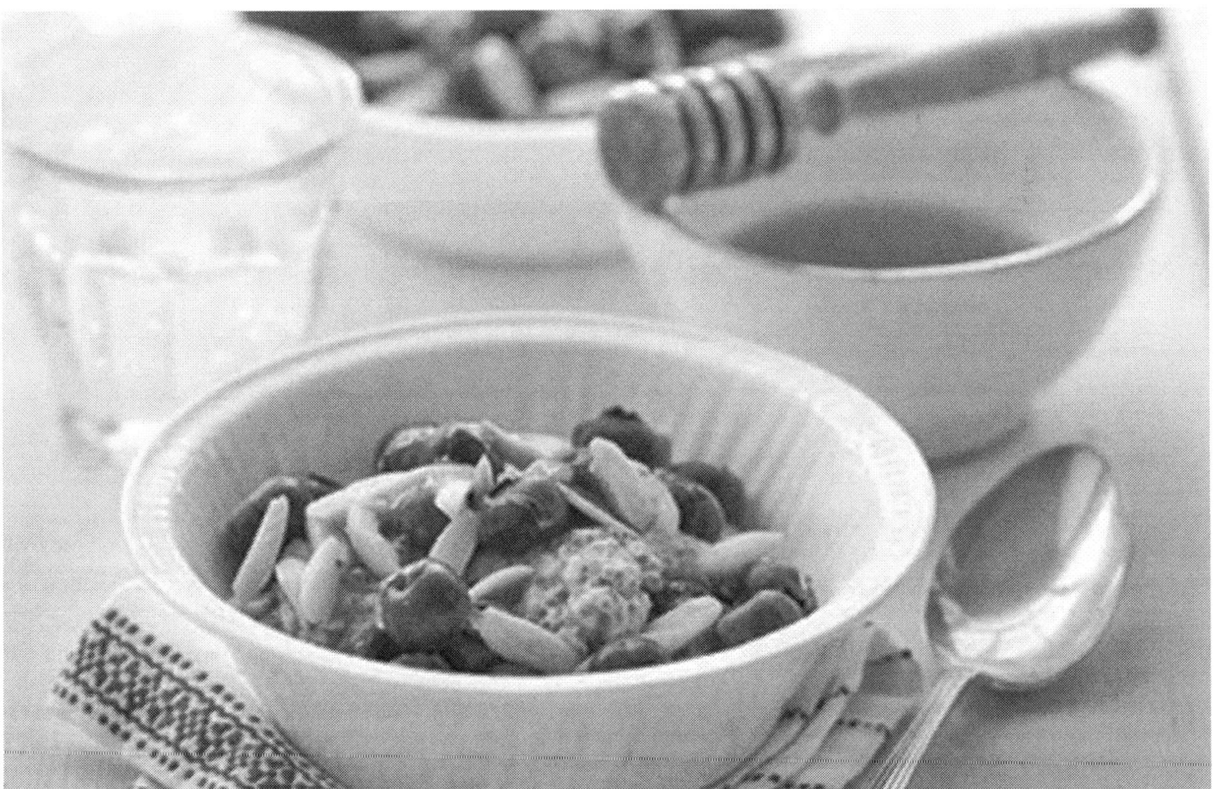

STRAWBERRIES AND COCONUT BREAKFAST

Cooking Difficulty: 2/10	Cooking Time: 12 minutes	Servings: 2

INGREDIENTS

- 3 tbsps. coconut flakes
- 2 tbsps. chopped strawberries
- 1 c. water
- 2/3 c. coconut milk
- ½ tsp. stevia

STEP 1

In your instant pot, mix strawberries with coconut flakes, water, milk, and stevia, stir, cover, and cook on High for 10 minutes.

STEP 2

Divide into 2 bowls and serve for breakfast.

STEP 3

Enjoy!

NUTRITIONAL INFORMATION

110 Calories, 5g Fat, 3g Carbs, 3g Protein

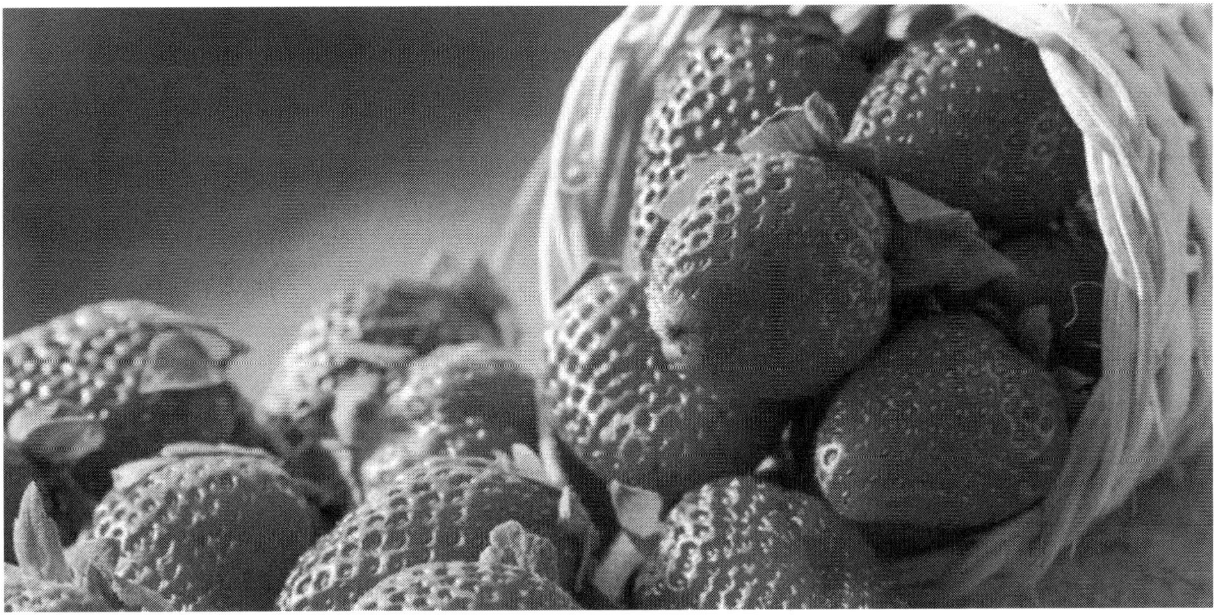

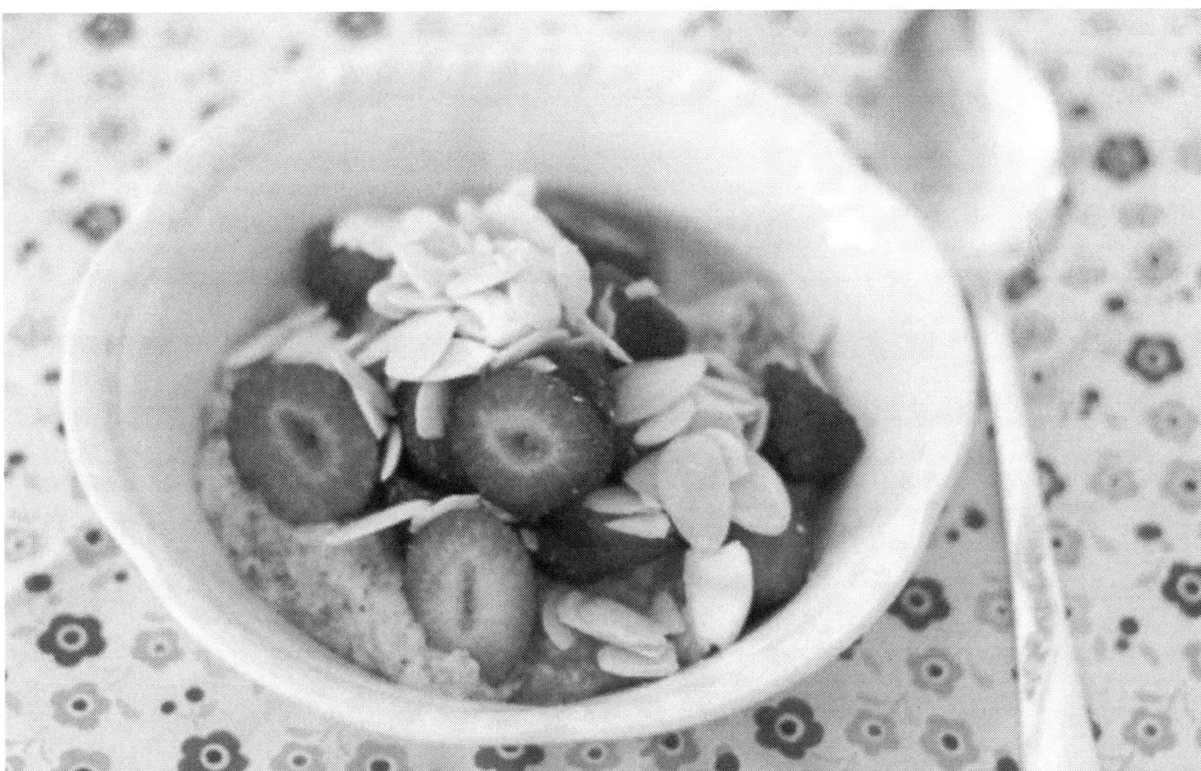

BUTTERED ASPARAGUS

STEP 1

In the center of a foil piece, place the asparagus and garlic and top with butter.

STEP 2

Curve the edges of foil slightly to avoid the leakage of butter.

STEP 3

In the bottom of the Instant Pot, arrange a steamer basket and pour 1 cup of water.

STEP 4

Place the asparagus on the steamer basket.

STEP 5

Close the lid, select STEAM, and cook for 8 minutes.

STEP 6

Press CANCEL and do a quick pressure release.

STEP 7

Remove the lid and transfer the asparagus onto serving plates.

STEP 8

Sprinkle with Parmesan and serve.

Cooking Difficulty: 2/10	Cooking Time: 10 minutes	Servings: 4

INGREDIENTS

- 1 lb. trimmed asparagus
- 3 garlic cloves
- 3 tbsps. softened butter
- 3 tbsps. grated parmesan cheese

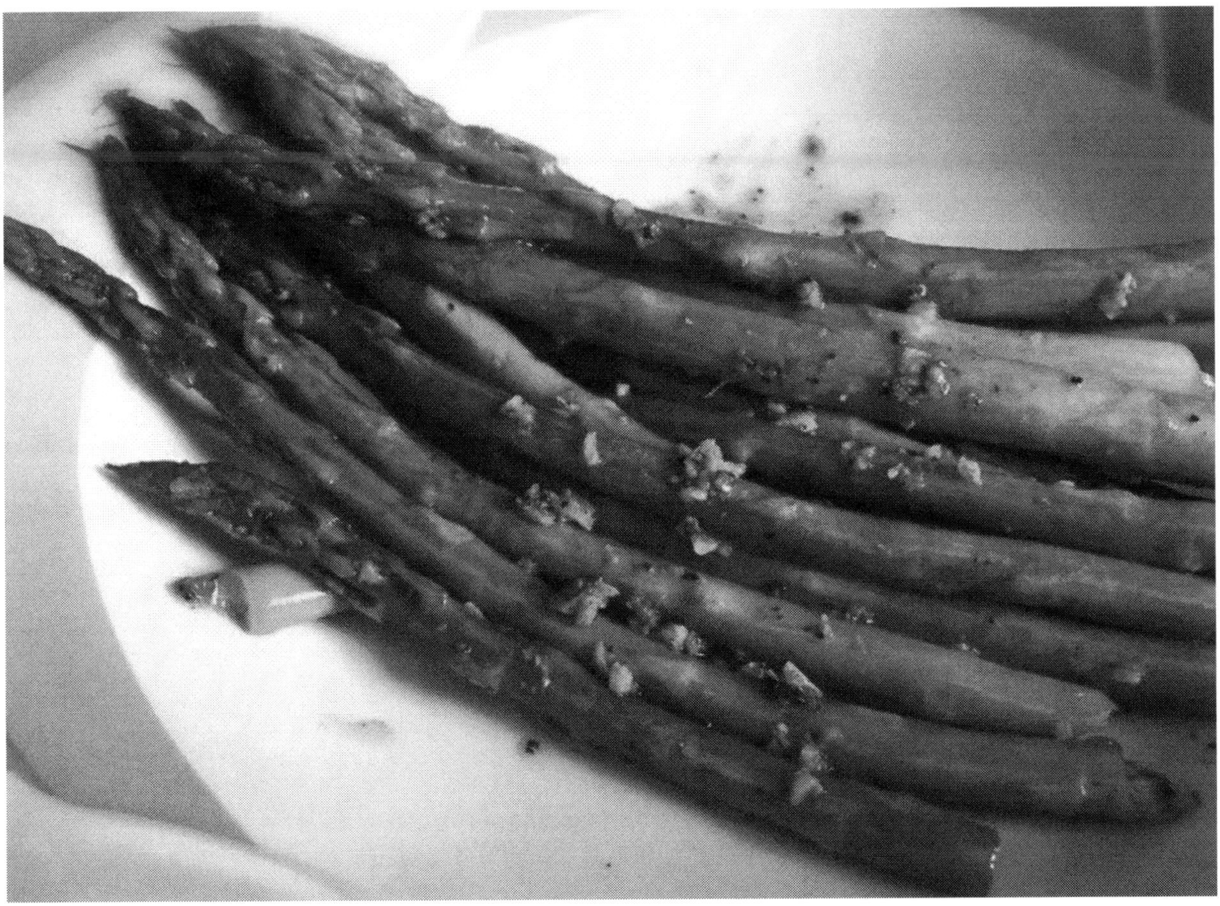

NUTRITIONAL INFORMATION

413 Calories, 37.1g Fat, 0.7g Carbs, 21g Protein

DIJON AND LEMON ARTICHOKES

Cooking Difficulty: 3/10	Cooking Time: 33 minutes	Servings: 4

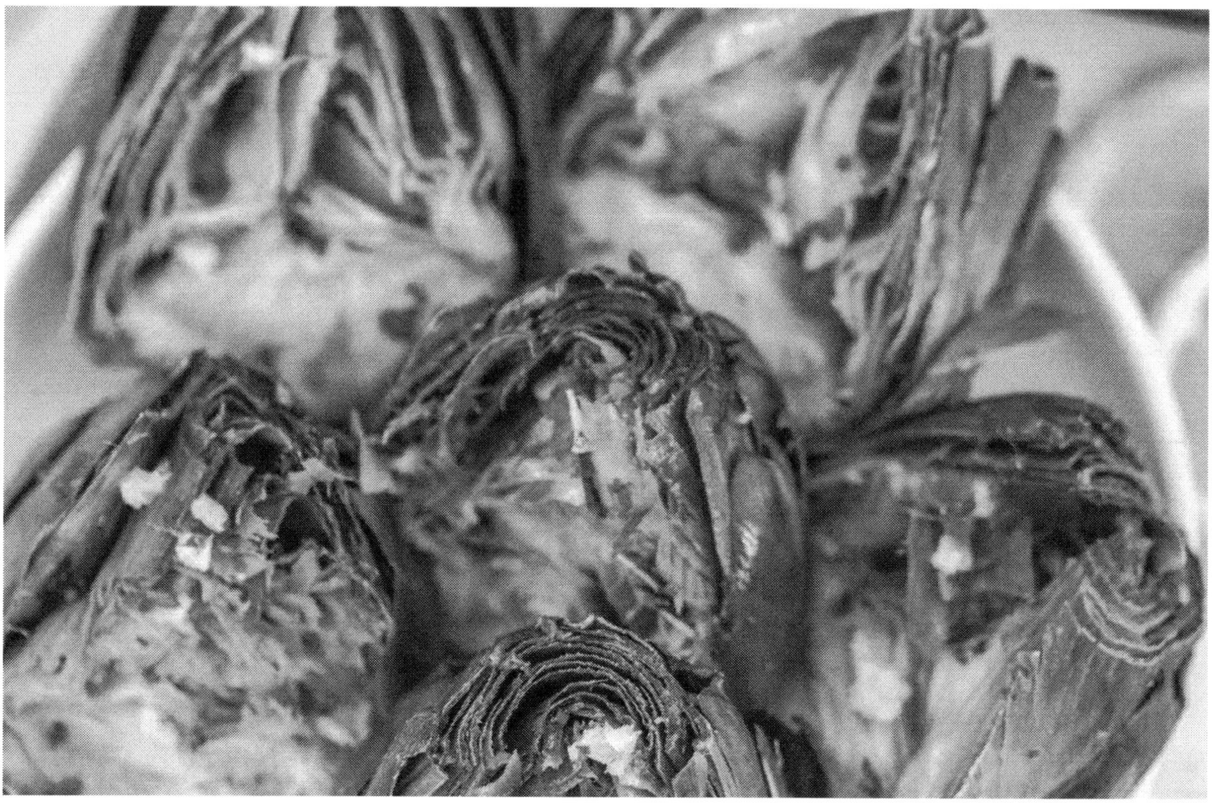

NUTRITIONAL INFORMATION

108 Calories, 7.5g Fat, 5.4g Carbs, 3.1g Protein

INGREDIENTS

- 1½ c. water
- 2 artichokes
- 1 lemon
- ¼ tsp. salt
- ¼ tsp. pepper
- 2 tbsps. dijon mustard
- 2 tbsps. olive oil
- 1 lemon wedge

STEP 1

Wash the artichokes well and trim them. Rub them with the lemon wedge.

STEP 2

Pour the water into the Instant Pot and lower the steamer basket.

STEP 3

Place the artichokes in the basket.

STEP 4

Close the lid and cook for 20 minutes on HIGH.

STEP 5

Do a natural pressure release, about 10 minutes. Quickly release the remaining pressure.

STEP 6

In a small bowl, mix together the lemon juice, mustard, olive oil, salt, and pepper.

STEP 7

Serve artichokes with the sauce.

STEP 8

Enjoy!

SOCKEYE SALMON

Cooking Difficulty: 2/10	Cooking Time: 10 minutes	Servings: 4

INGREDIENTS

- 4 sockeye salmon fillets
- 1 tsp. dijon mustard
- ¼ tsp. minced garlic
- 1 tbsp. lemon juice
- ¼ tsp. onion powder
- ¼ tsp. lemon pepper
- ½ tsp. garlic powder
- ¼ tsp. salt
- 2 tbsps. olive oil
- 1½ c. water

STEP 1

In a bowl, combine the mustard, garlic, lemon juice, onion powder, lemon pepper, garlic powder, salt, and olive oil. Brush the spice mixture over the salmon fillets.

STEP 2

Pour the water into the Instant Pot. Lower the trivet.

STEP 3

Place the salmon fillets on the rack and close the lid.

STEP 4

Set the Instant Pot to MANUAL and cook at low pressure for 7 minutes.

STEP 5

Release the pressure quickly. Serve and enjoy!

NUTRITIONAL INFORMATION

353 Calories, 25g Fat, 0.6g Carbs, 40.6g Protein

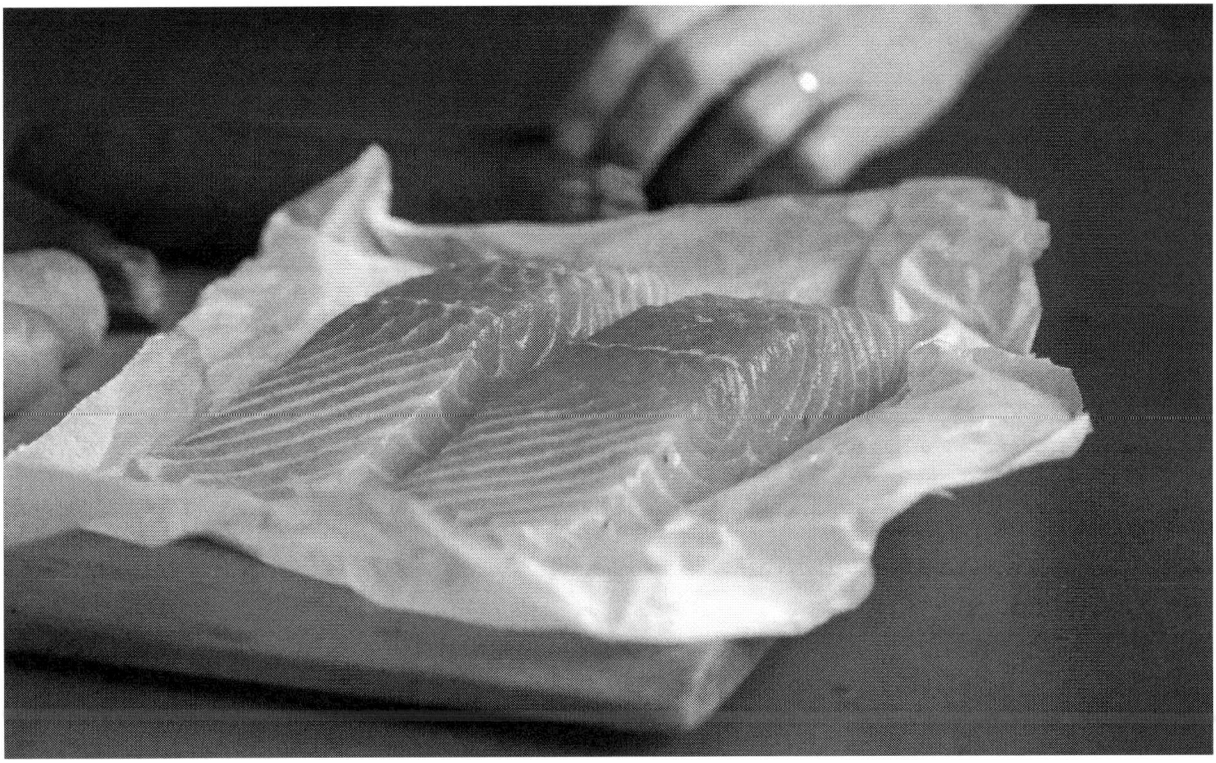

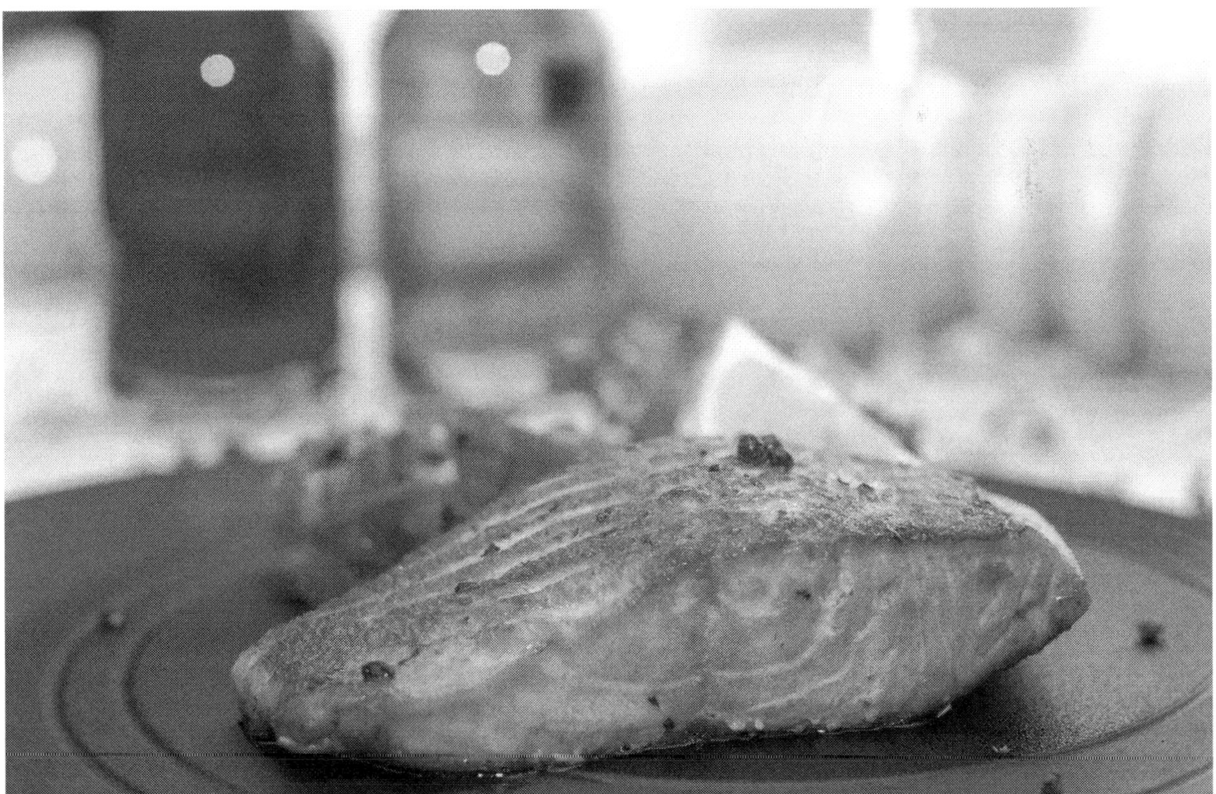

TENDER BEEF POT ROAST

STEP 1
Heat 1 tbsp. of olive oil in the Instant Pot on SAUTÉ.

STEP 2
Add the beef and sear it on all sides until browned, about 5 minutes in total. Transfer to a plate.

STEP 3
Heat the remaining oil in the Instant Pot and add the onions, celery, and pepper. Cook for a few minutes, until soft.

STEP 4
Add garlic and cook for 30 seconds.

STEP 5
Return the meat to the pot.

STEP 6
In a bowl, whisk together the vinegar, broth, and Italian Seasoning. Pour the mixture over the beef.

STEP 7
Close the lid and cook on HIGH for 40 minutes.

STEP 8
Release the pressure naturally.

STEP 9
Serve and enjoy!

Cooking Difficulty: 4/10	Cooking Time: 48 minutes	Servings: 6

INGREDIENTS

- 1 sliced onion
- 2 tbsps. minced garlic
- 2½ lbs. beef roast
- 2 tbsps. sugar-free steak sauce
- 2 chopped celery stalks
- 1 chopped bell pepper
- 2 tbsps. olive oil
- 1 c. beef broth
- 1 tbsp. balsamic vinegar
- 1½ tbsps. italian seasoning

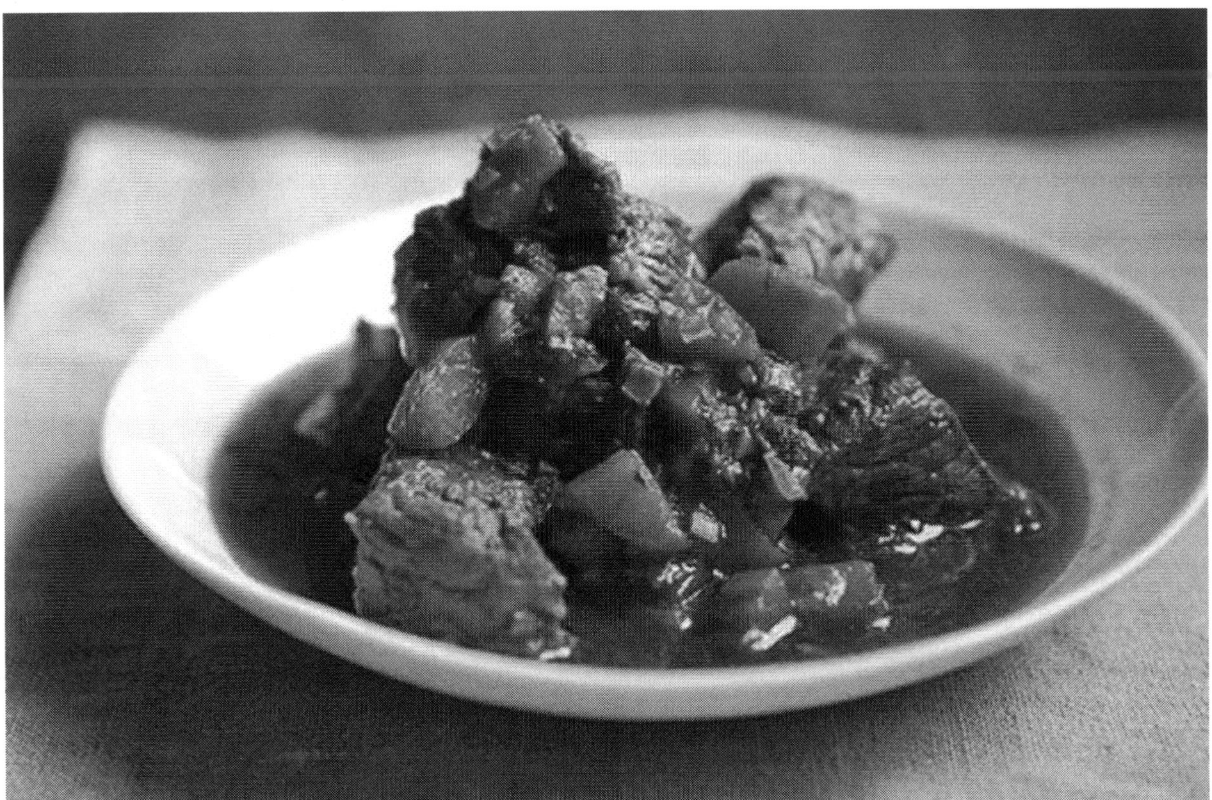

NUTRITIONAL INFORMATION

603 Calories, 40.4g Fat, 4.5g Carbs, 51.7g Protein

BALSAMIC-GLAZED PORK LOIN

Cooking Difficulty: 3/10	Cooking Time: 66 minutes	Servings: 4

INGREDIENTS

- 1 minced garlic clove
- 1 tsp. sage
- 2 lbs. pork loin
- ½ c. beef broth
- ½ tsp. pepper

glaze:

- 1 tbsp. arrowroot
- ¼ c. balsamic vinegar
- ½ c. swerve
- 2 tbsps. coconut aminos
- ½ c. water

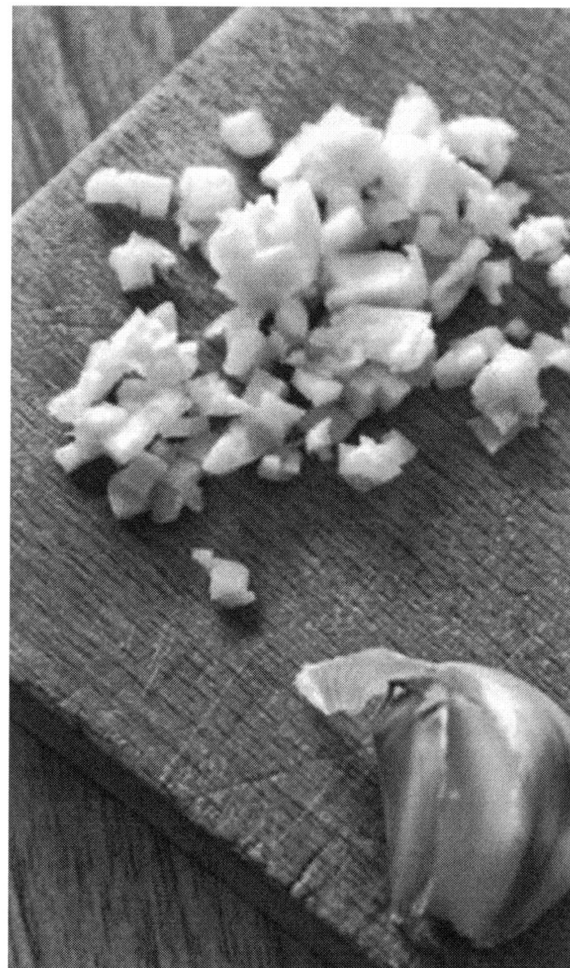

NUTRITIONAL INFORMATION

568 Calories, 31.8g Fat, 12.5g Carbs, 42.8g Protein

STEP 1

Rub the pork with sage, pepper, and garlic. Place it inside the Instant Pot and pour the broth over.

STEP 2

Close lid tightly and set the IP to MANUAL. Cook on HIGH for 1 hour.

STEP 3

Release the pressure naturally for 10 minutes. Quickly release the remaining pressure.

STEP 4

Meanwhile, whisk together the glaze ingredients.

STEP 5

You can either brush the mixture over the pork loin and sear on SAUTÉ for a few minutes or shred the meat, pour the sauce over and cook on SAUTÉ for 2-3 minutes. Serve and enjoy!

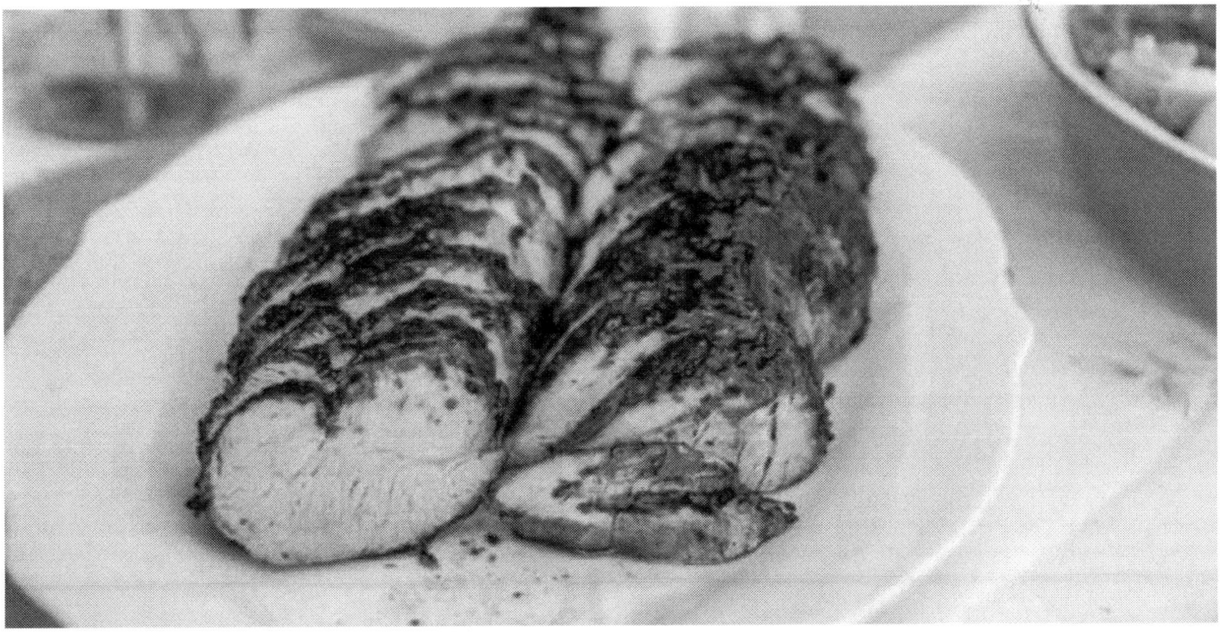

FRENCH ONION PORK CHOPS

Cooking Difficulty: 3/10	Cooking Time: 27 minutes	Servings: 4

INGREDIENTS

- 4 pork chops
- 10 oz. french onion soup
- ½ c. sour cream
- 10 oz. chicken broth

STEP 1

Place pork chops in the IP and pour the broth over.

STEP 2

Close the lid and cook on HIGH for 12 minutes.

STEP 3

Release the pressure naturally.

STEP 4

Whisk together the sour cream and French onion soup and pour the mixture over the pork.

STEP 5

Set the Instant Pot to SAUTÉ and cook for about 6–8 minutes.

STEP 6

Serve and enjoy!

NUTRITIONAL INFORMATION

365 Calories, 26.9g Fat, 6.9g Carbs, 21.5g Protein

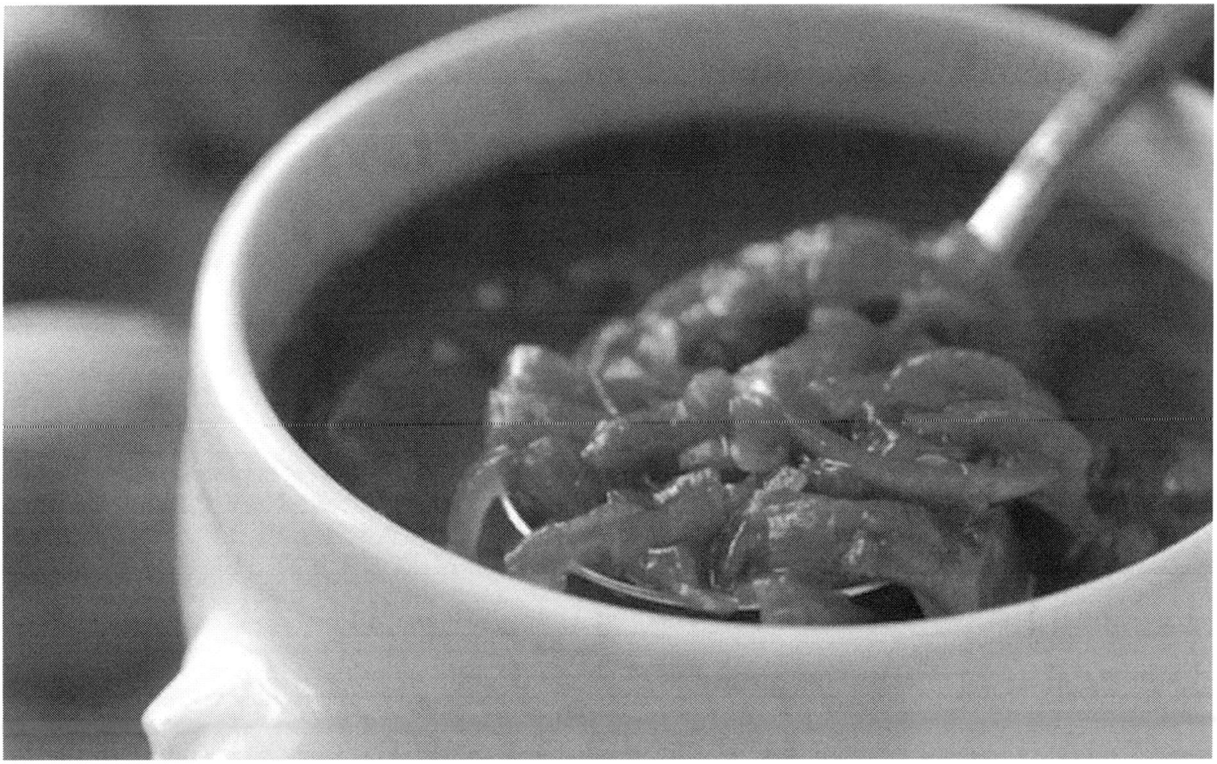

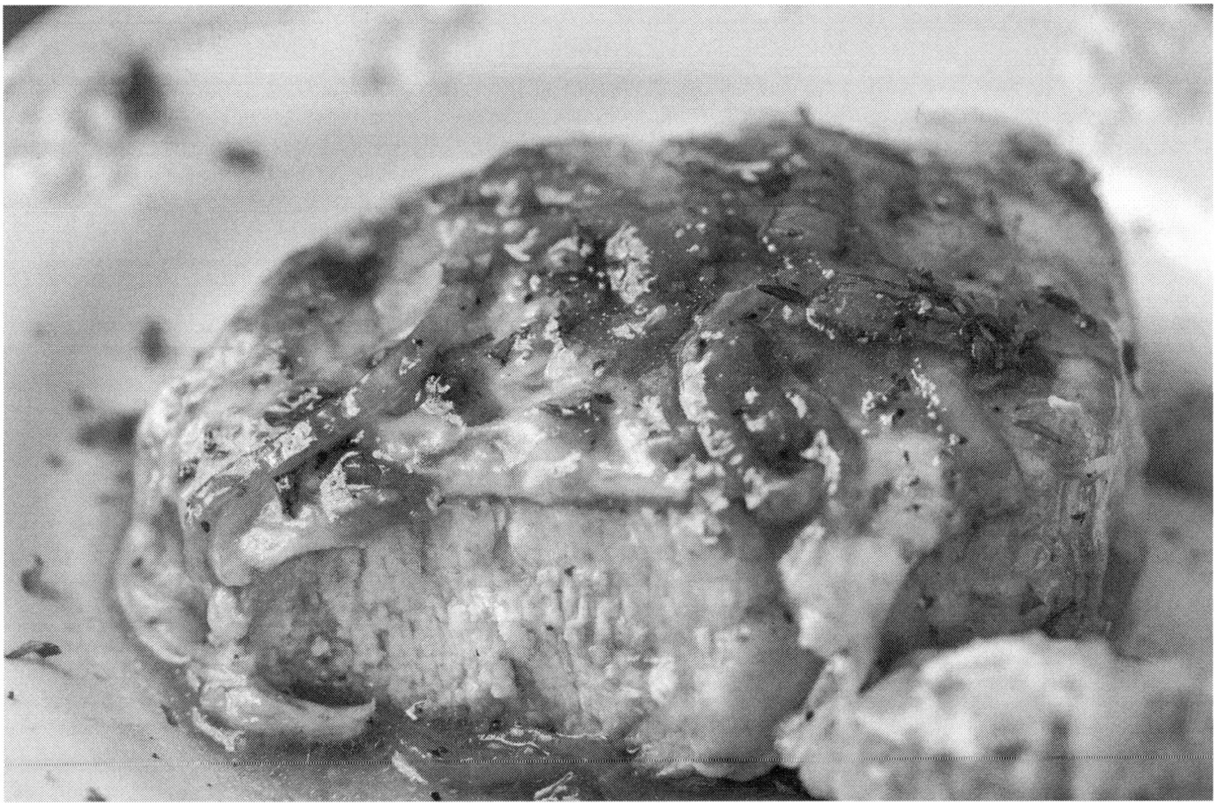

POMODORO SOUP WITH BASIL

Cooking Difficulty: 3/10	Cooking Time: 20 minutes	Servings: 6

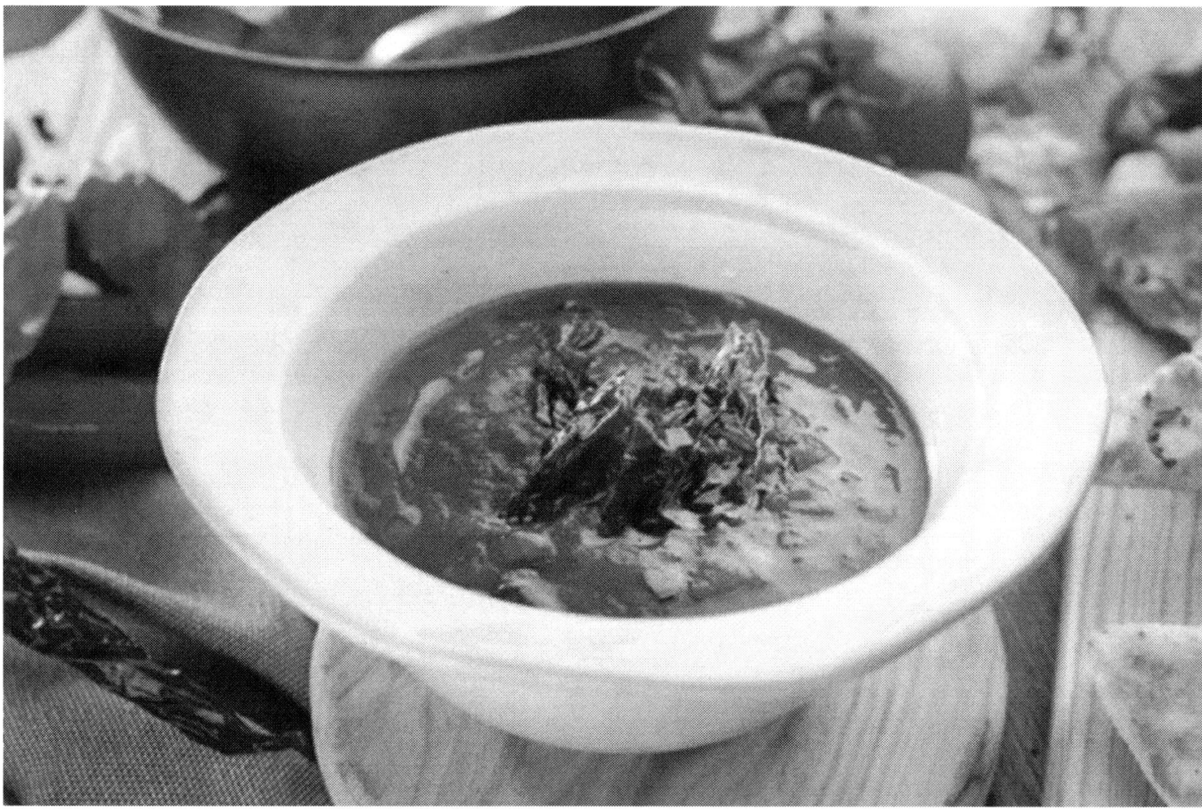

NUTRITIONAL INFORMATION

196 Calories, 13.2g Fat, 8.8g Carbs, 9.4g Protein

INGREDIENTS

- 2 tbsps. olive oil
- ½ diced onion
- 2 tbsps. tomato paste
- 3 c. vegetable broth
- 28 oz. diced tomatoes
- chopped basil
- 1 tsp. balsamic vinegar
- ½ c. shredded cheddar cheese

STEP 1

Set your Instant Pot on SAUTÉ and heat the oil in it. Add the onions and sauté for 3–4 minutes.

STEP 2

Stir in the tomato paste and cook for 30–60 seconds.

STEP 3

Pour the broth over and stir in the tomatoes.

STEP 4

Close the lid and cook on SOUP for 10 minutes.

STEP 5

Release the pressure naturally.

STEP 6

Stir in half of the basil and the balsamic vinegar. Use a hand blender to blend the mixture until smooth.

STEP 7

Top with the remaining basil and serve. Enjoy!

FISH STEW

Cooking Difficulty: 2/10	Cooking Time: 10 minutes	Servings: 6

INGREDIENTS

- 3 c. fish stock
- 1 diced onion
- 1 c. chopped broccoli
- 2 c. chopped celery stalks
- 1½ c. diced cauliflower
- 1 sliced carrot
- 1 lb. chopped white fish fillets
- 1 c. heavy cream
- 1 bay leaf
- 2 tbsps. butter
- ¼ tsp. pepper
- ½ tsp. salt
- ¼ tsp. garlic powder

STEP 1

Set your Instant Pot to SAUTÉ and melt the butter in it. Add onion and carrots (if using), and cook for 3 minutes.

STEP 2

Stir in the remaining ingredients.

STEP 3

Close the lid and hit MANUAL. Cook for 4 minutes on HIGH.

STEP 4

Do a natural pressure release. Discard the bay leaf.

STEP 5

Serve and enjoy!

NUTRITIONAL INFORMATION

294 Calories, 18g Fat, 6.1g Carbs, 24.2g Protein

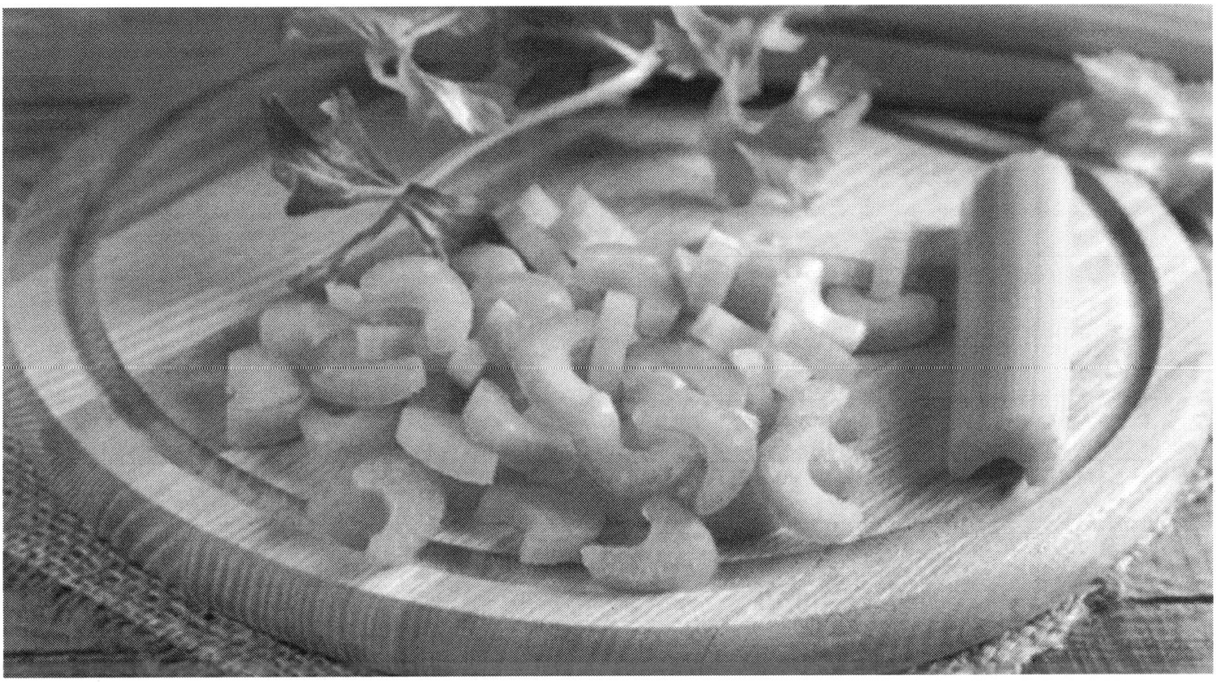

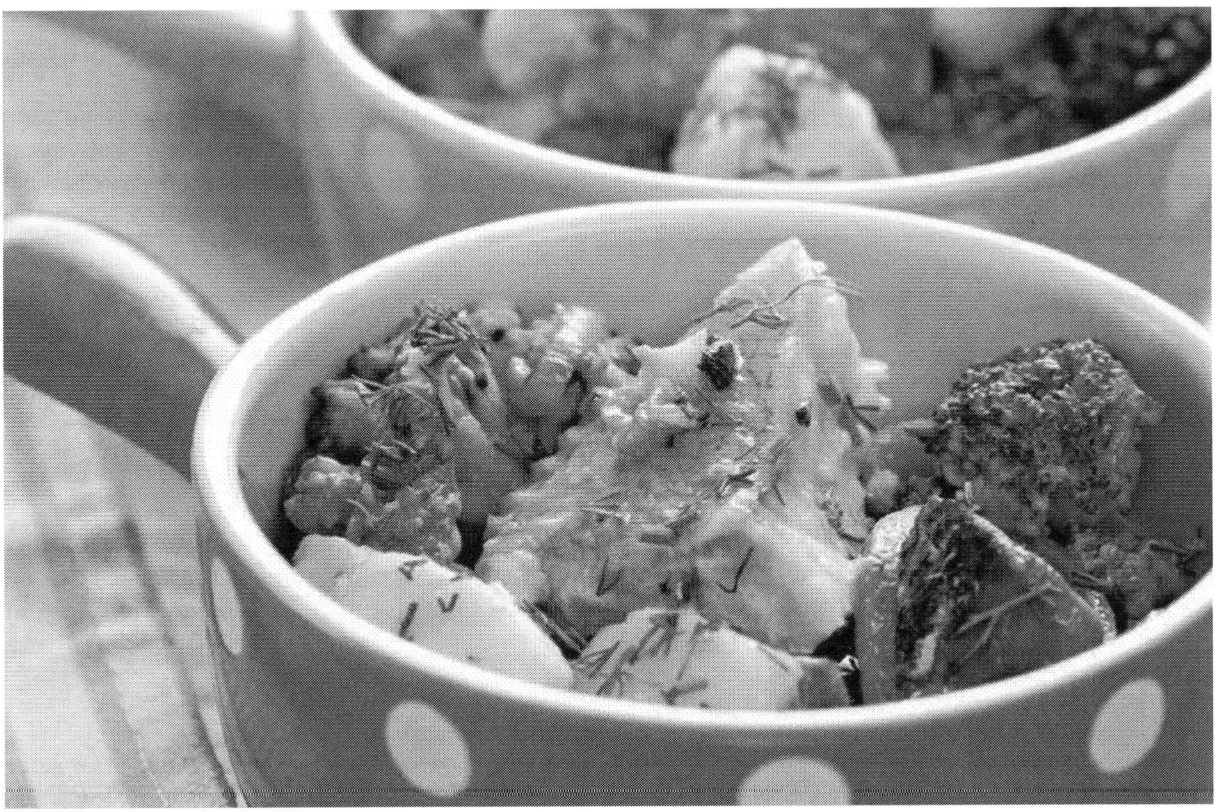

KETO CHILI

INGREDIENTS

- 2 tbsps. olive oil
- ½ tsp. cumin
- 2 tbsps. tomato paste
- 2 lbs. ground beef
- 1 c. diced tomatoes
- 1 tsp. chili powder
- 1 diced onion
- 1 c. beef broth
- 1 tsp. minced garlic
- salt
- pepper

STEP 1
Set the Instant Pot to SAUTÉ and heat the olive oil in it.

STEP 2
Cook the onions for about 2 minutes. Add garlic and cook for 1 minute.

STEP 3
Add the beef and cook until it is browned, breaking it with a spatula.

STEP 4
Stir in the tomato paste and spices and cook for 1 more minute.

STEP 5
Stir in the broth and tomatoes.

STEP 6
Close the lid and cook for 30 minutes on MEAT/STEW.

STEP 7
Do a quick pressure release.

STEP 8
Serve and enjoy!

Cooking Difficulty: 3/10	Cooking Time: 38 minutes	Servings: 4

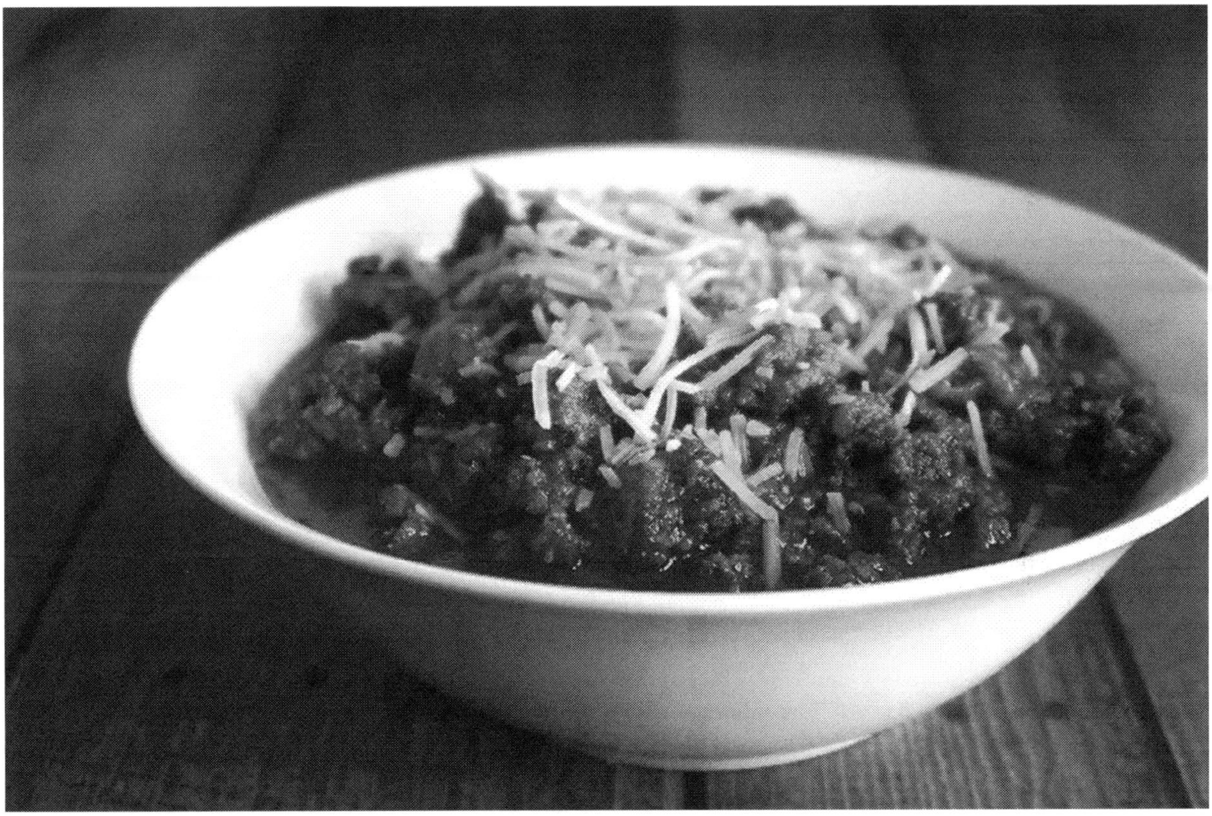

NUTRITIONAL INFORMATION

505 Calories, 33.5g Fat, 5.1g Carbs, 42.7g Protein

CHILI TOMATO PORK STEW

STEP 1

Rinse the pork shoulder, pat dry. Cut into chunks.

STEP 2

Press the Sauté button on Instant Pot. Heat the coconut oil.

STEP 3

Add onion, garlic. Sweat for 1 minute. Add pork shoulder. Brown on all sides.

STEP 4

Add mushrooms, bell peppers. Sauté until vegetables have softened.

STEP 5

Press the Keep Warm/Cancel button to stop Sauté mode.

STEP 6

Add the rest of the ingredients. Stir well.

STEP 7

Close and seal lid. Press the Soup button. Cook for 30 minutes.

STEP 8

When the timer beeps, quick-release, or naturally release pressure. Open lid carefully. Stir ingredients.

STEP 9

Serve.

Cooking Difficulty: 4/10	Cooking Time: 38 minutes	Servings: 4

INGREDIENTS

- 1 lb. pork shoulder
- 1 diced red onion
- 2 minced garlic cloves
- 2 tbsps. coconut oil
- 6 oz. sliced mushrooms
- 1 chopped green bell pepper
- 1 chopped red bell pepper
- 4 c. beef broth
- 1 tbsp. lime juice
- ½ c. tomato paste
- 2 tsps. chili powder
- 2 tsps. ground cumin
- 1 tbsp. chopped cilantro
- 1 tsp. smoked paprika
- 1 tsp. salt
- 1 tsp. black pepper

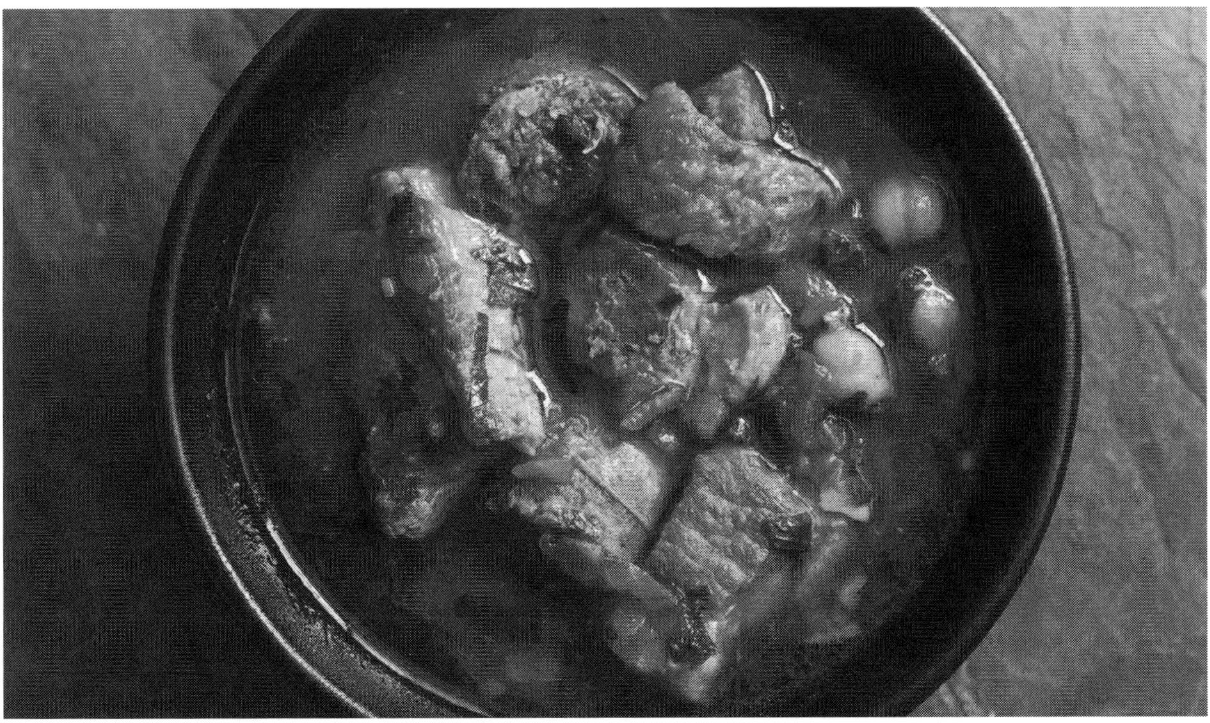

NUTRITIONAL INFORMATION

350 Calories, 28g Fat, 10g Carbs, 20g Protein

CELERIAC FRIES

Cooking Difficulty: 2/10	Cooking Time: 9 minutes	Servings: 2

INGREDIENTS

- 2 big peeled celeriac
- 1 c. water
- salt
- ¼ tsp. baking soda
- olive oil

STEP 1

Put the water in your instant pot, add salt and the baking soda and the steamer basket, add celeriac fries inside, cover, cook on High for 4 minutes, drain and transfer them to a bowl.

STEP 2

Place olive oil on a pan and heat over medium-high heat, add celeriac fries, cook until they are golden on all sides, drain grease, transfer them to plates and serve as a side dish.

STEP 3

Enjoy!

NUTRITIONAL INFORMATION

182 Calories, 5g Fat, 7g Carbs, 10g Protein

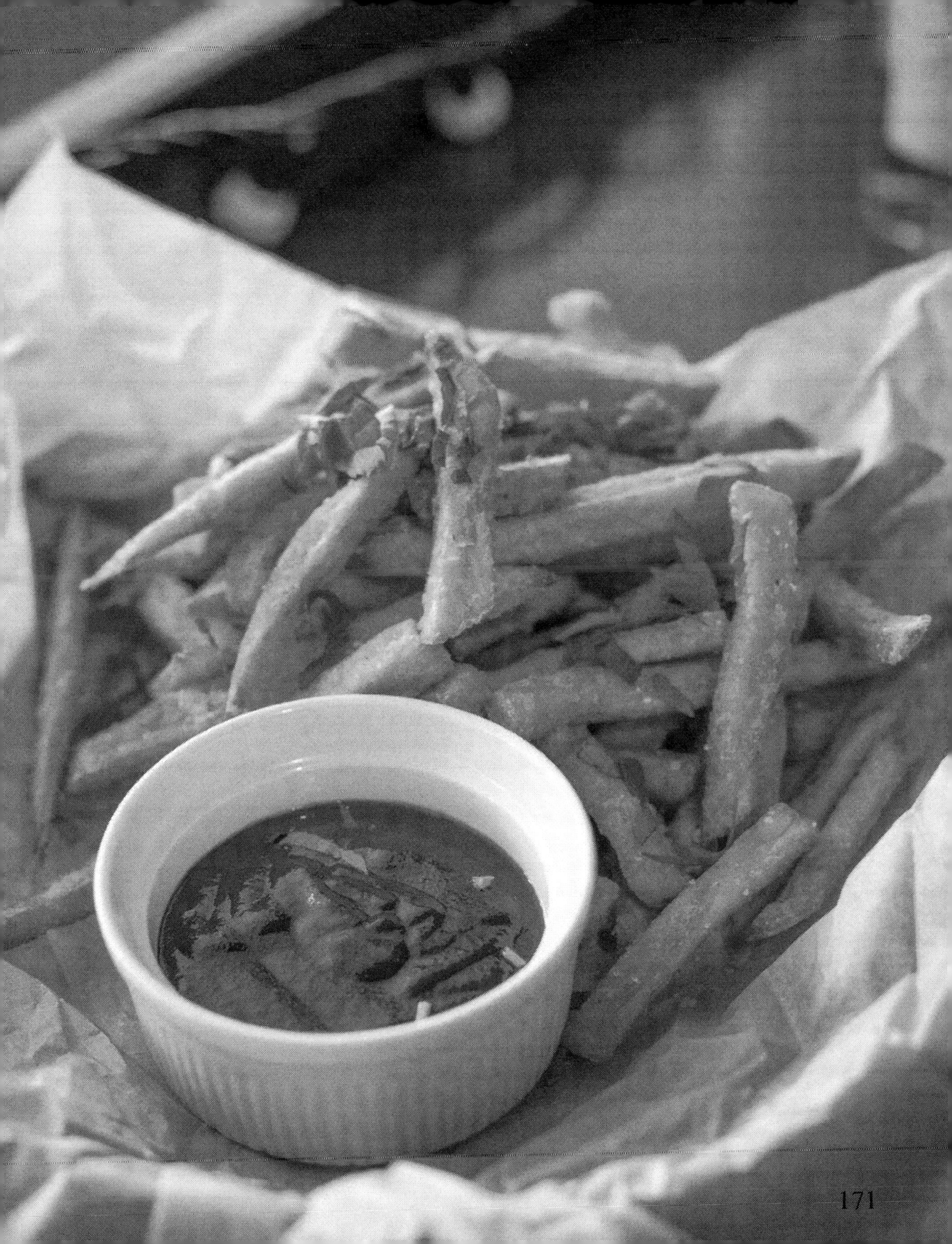

KALE AND ALMONDS

Cooking Difficulty: 2/10	Cooking Time: 8 minutes	Servings: 4

INGREDIENTS

- 1 c. water
- 1 big kale bunch, chopped
- 1 tbsp. balsamic vinegar
- 1/3 c. toasted almonds
- 3 minced garlic cloves
- 1 small chopped yellow onion
- 2 tbsps. olive oil

STEP 1
Set your instant pot on sauté mode, add oil, heat it up, add onion, stir and cook for 3 minutes.

STEP 2
Add garlic, water and kale, stir, cover and cook on High for 4 minutes.

STEP 3
Add salt, pepper, vinegar, and almonds, toss well, divide between plates and serve as a side dish.

STEP 4
Enjoy!

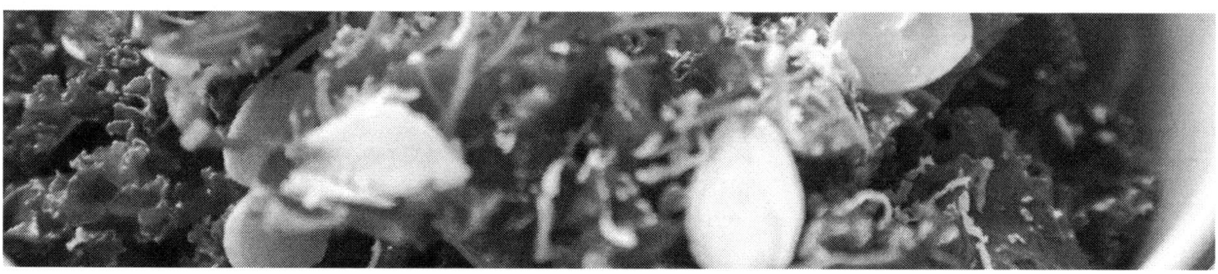

NUTRITIONAL INFORMATION
140 Calories, 6g Fat, 5g Carbs, 3g Protein

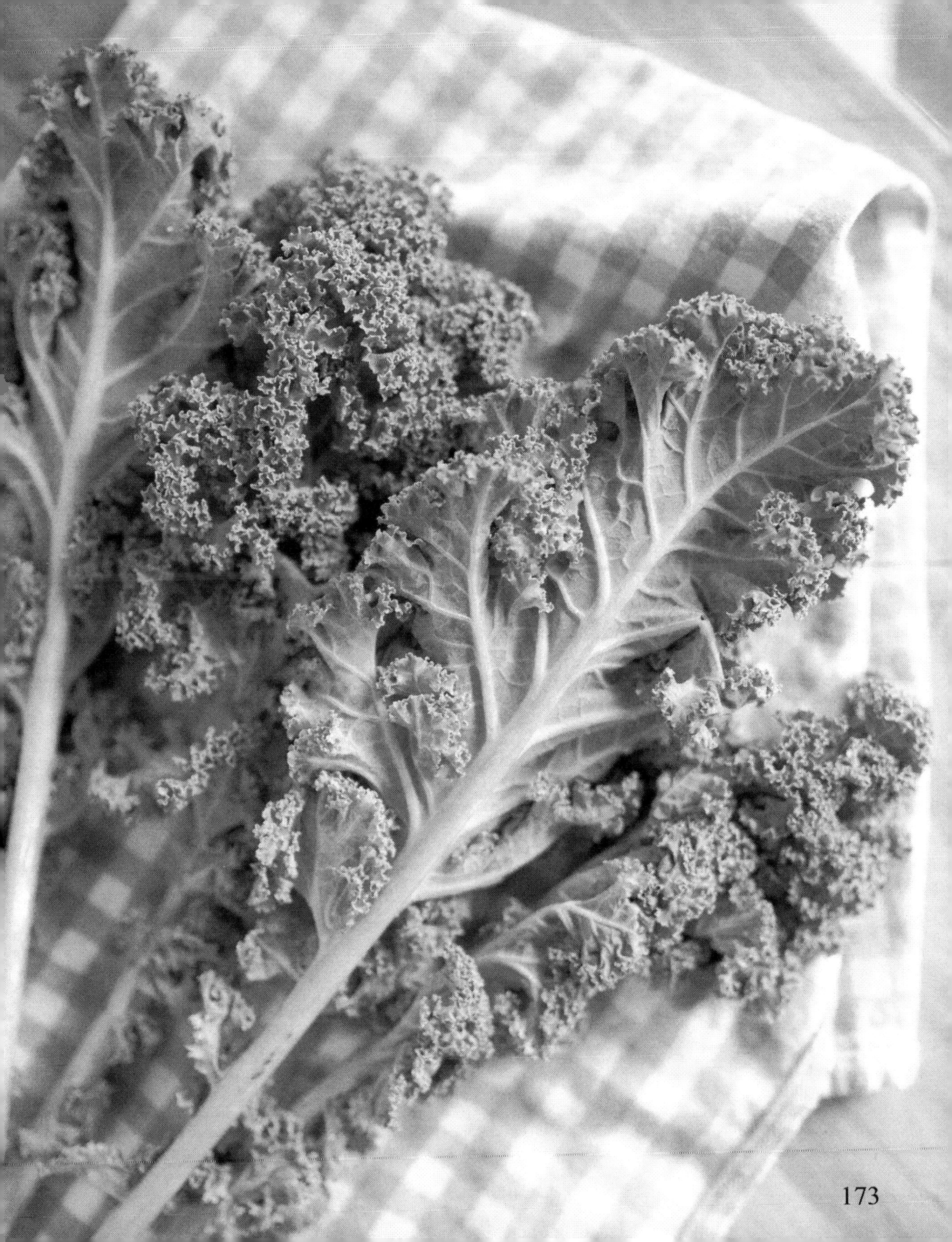

RED CHARD AND OLIVES

Cooking Difficulty: 2/10	Cooking Time: 5 minutes	Servings: 4

INGREDIENTS

- 2 tbsps. olive oil
- 1 bunch chopped red chard
- 3 tbsps. veggie stock
- 2 tbsps. capers
- 1 chopped yellow onion
- juice of 1 lemon
- salt
- black pepper
- 1 tsp. stevia
- ¼ c. chopped kalamata olives

STEP 1

Set your instant pot on sauté mode, add oil, heat it up, add onion, stir and cook for 2 minutes.

STEP 2

Add stevia, olives, chard, salt, pepper, and stock, stir, cover, and cook on High for 3 minutes.

STEP 3

Add capers and lemon juice, stir, divide between plates and serve as a side dish.

STEP 4

Enjoy!

NUTRITIONAL INFORMATION

123 Calories, 4g Fat, 4g Carbs, 5g Protein

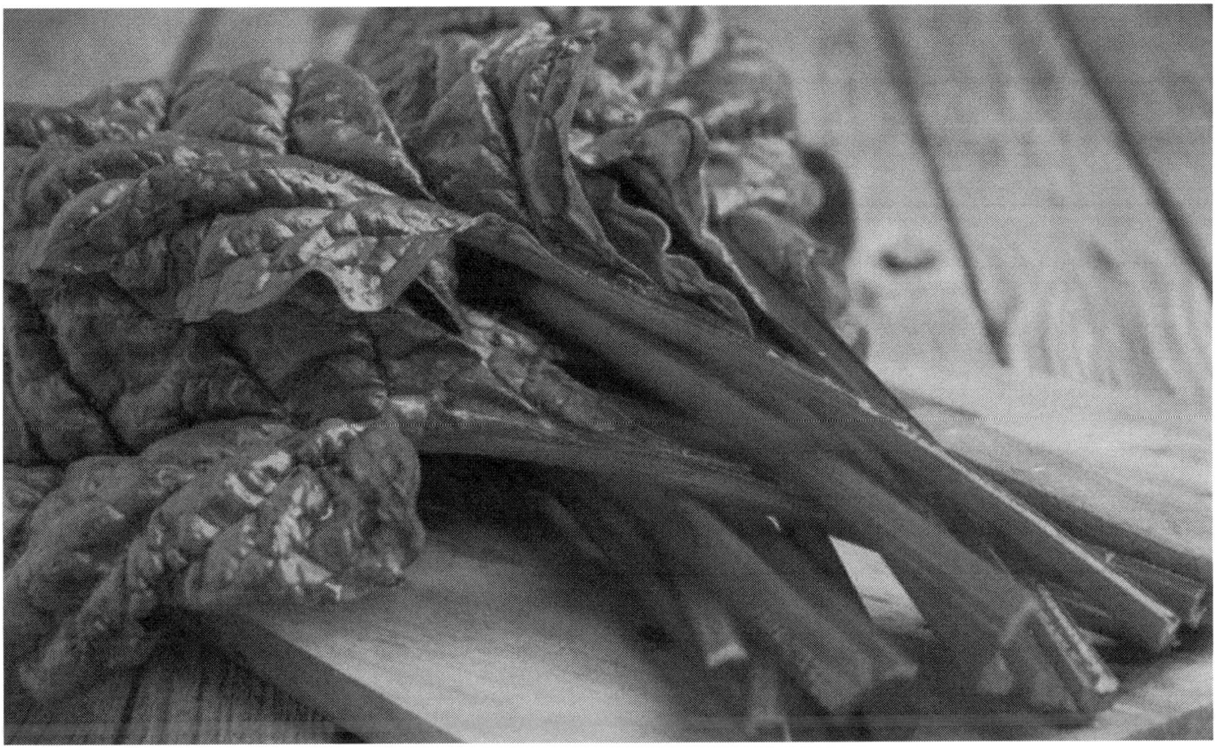

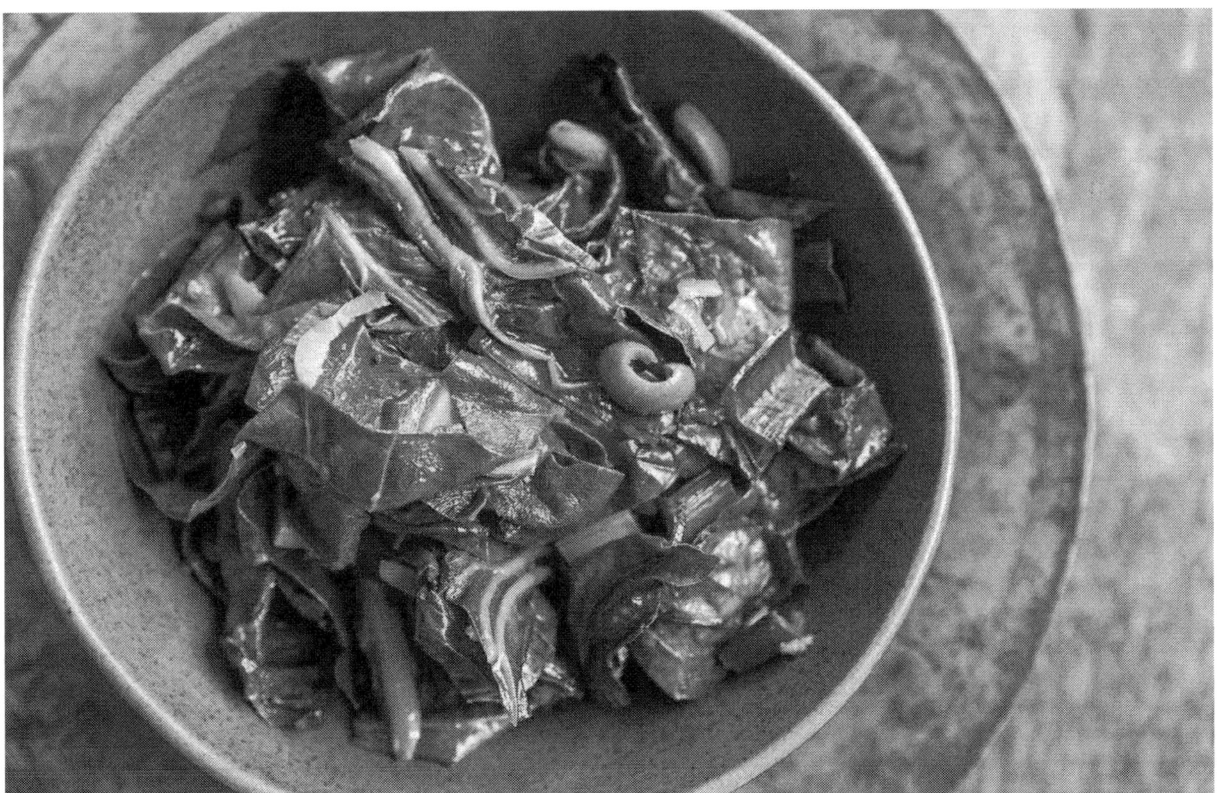

CHERRY TOMATO MACKEREL

Cooking Difficulty: 2/10	Cooking Time: 10 minutes	Servings: 4

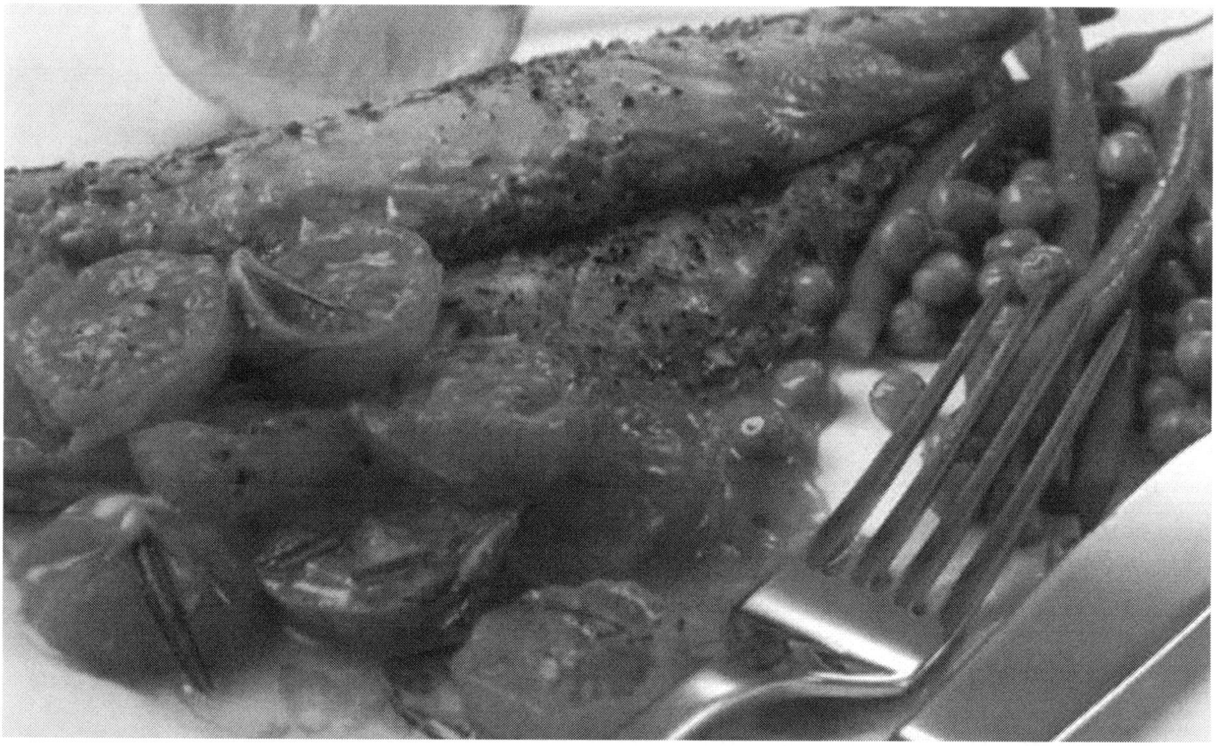

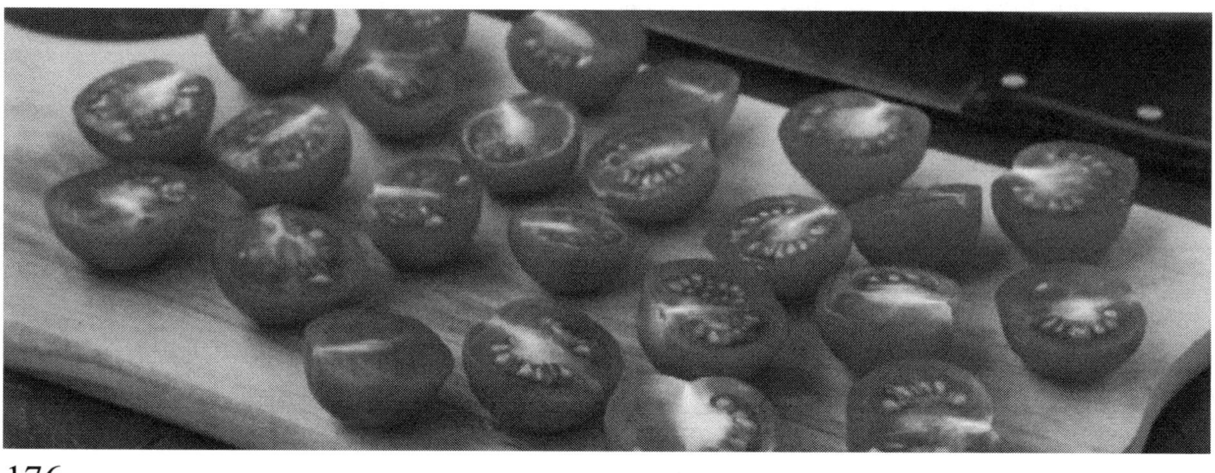

INGREDIENTS

- 4 mackerel fillets
- ¼ tsp. onion powder
- ¼ tsp. lemon pepper
- ¼ tsp. garlic powder
- ¼ tsp. salt
- 2 c. cherry tomatoes
- 3 tbsps. melted butter
- 1½ c. water
- 1 tbsp. black olives

STEP 1

Grease a baking dish that fits inside the Instant Pot with some cooking spray.

STEP 2

Arrange the cherry tomatoes at the bottom of the dish. Top with the mackerel fillets and sprinkle with all of the spices. Drizzle the melted butter over.

STEP 3

Pour water into Instant Pot and lower the trivet.

STEP 4

Place the baking dish on the trivet. Close the lid.

STEP 5

Set the Instant Pot to MANUAL and cook at low pressure for 7 minutes.

STEP 6

Do a quick pressure release.

STEP 7

Serve and enjoy!

NUTRITIONAL INFORMATION

325 Calories, 24.5g Fat, 2.7g Carbs, 21.9g Protein

SOUTHERN COLLARD GREENS

Cooking Difficulty: 2/10	Cooking Time: 13 minutes	Servings: 5

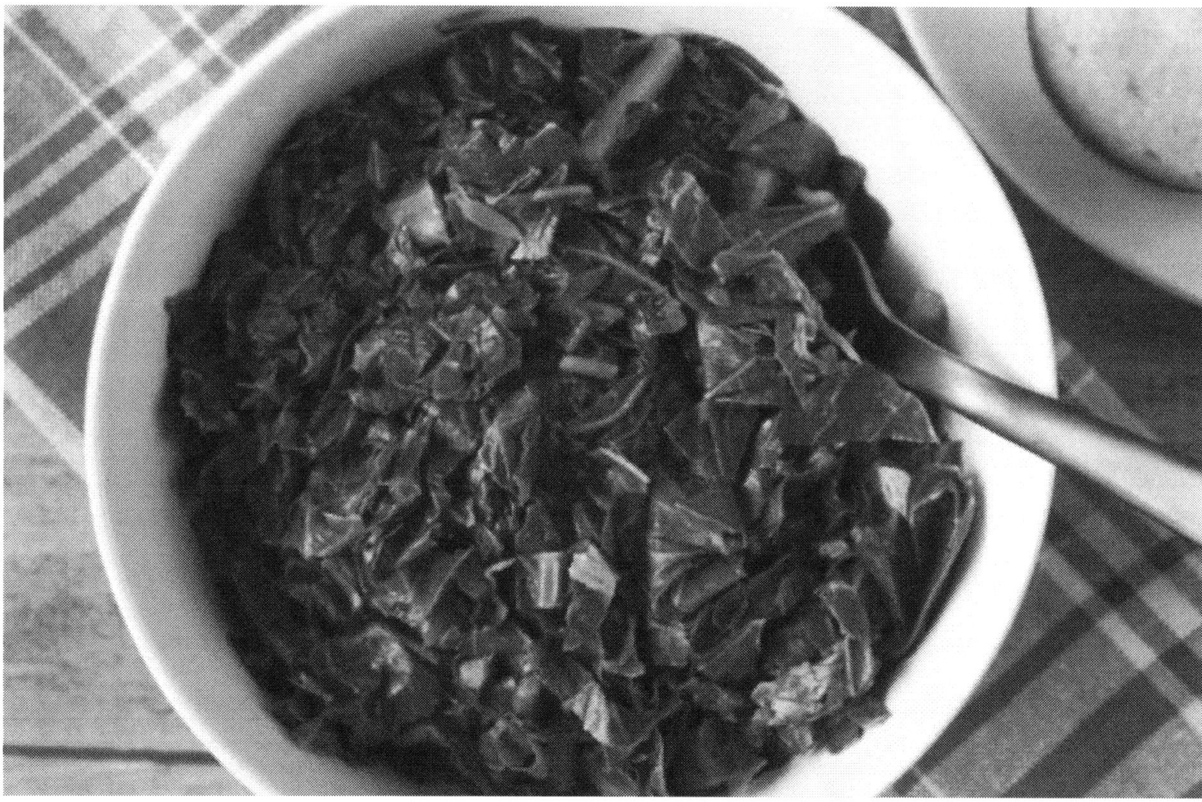

NUTRITIONAL INFORMATION

106 Calories, 6.9g Fat, 2.38g Carbs, 4.3g Protein

INGREDIENTS

- 2 bunches collard greens
- 2 tbsps. olive oil
- 1 yellow onion
- 3 minced garlic cloves
- red pepper flakes
- 1 c. water
- salt

STEP 1

Remove the tough stems of collard greens and then cut them into thin strands.

STEP 2

Place olive oil in the Instant Pot and select “Sauté.” Then add the onion and cook for about 4-5 minutes.

STEP 3

Add the garlic and red pepper flakes and cook for about 1 minute.

STEP 4

Select the “Cancel” and stir in collard greens and water.

STEP 5

While the lid is secured, set the pressure valve to the “Seal” position.

STEP 6

Select “Manual” and cook for 3 minutes under “High Pressure.”

STEP 7

Select the “Cancel” and carefully do a Quick Release.

STEP 8

Remove the lid and stir in salt. Serve hot.

SNACKS & DESSERTS

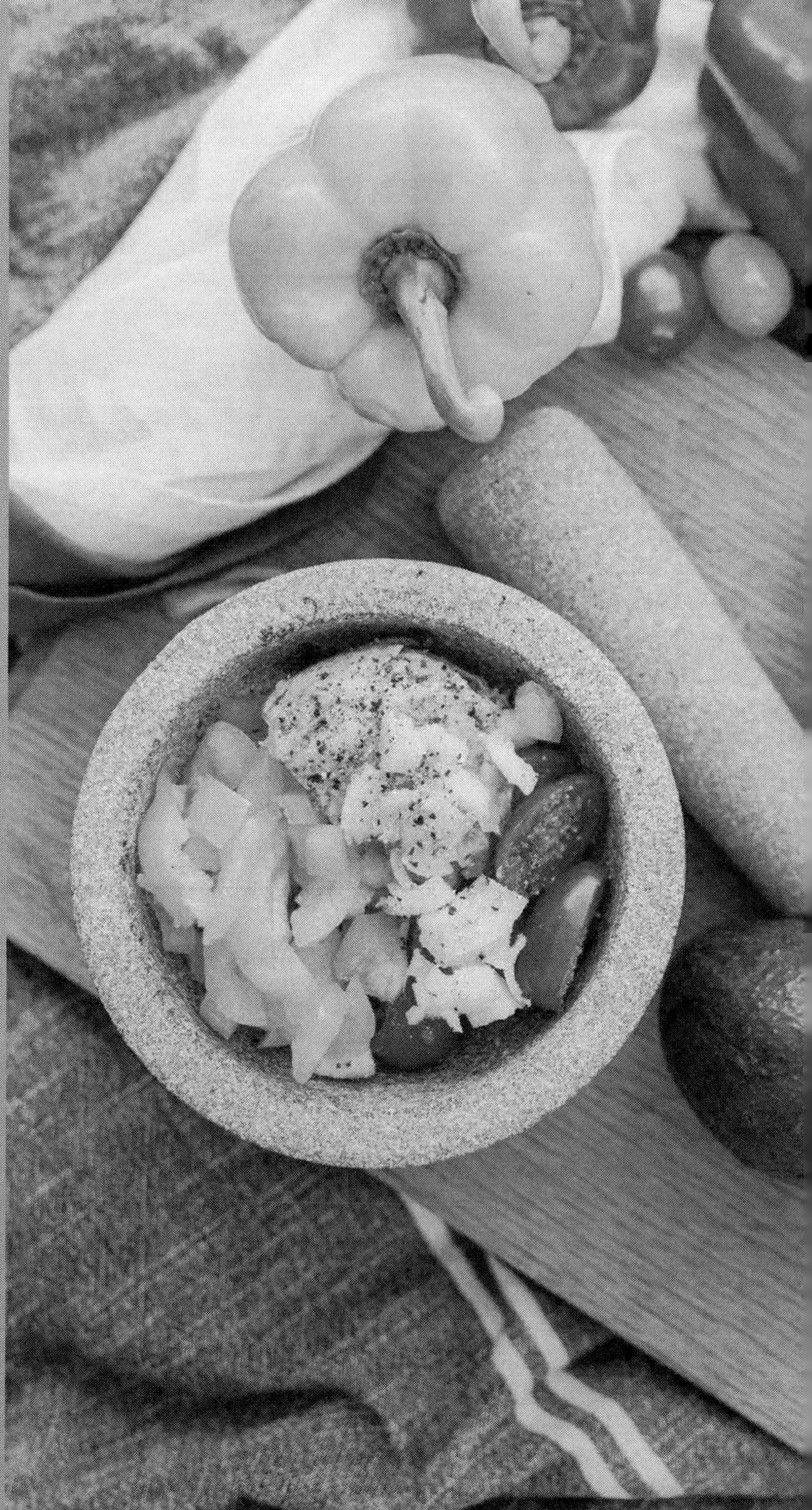

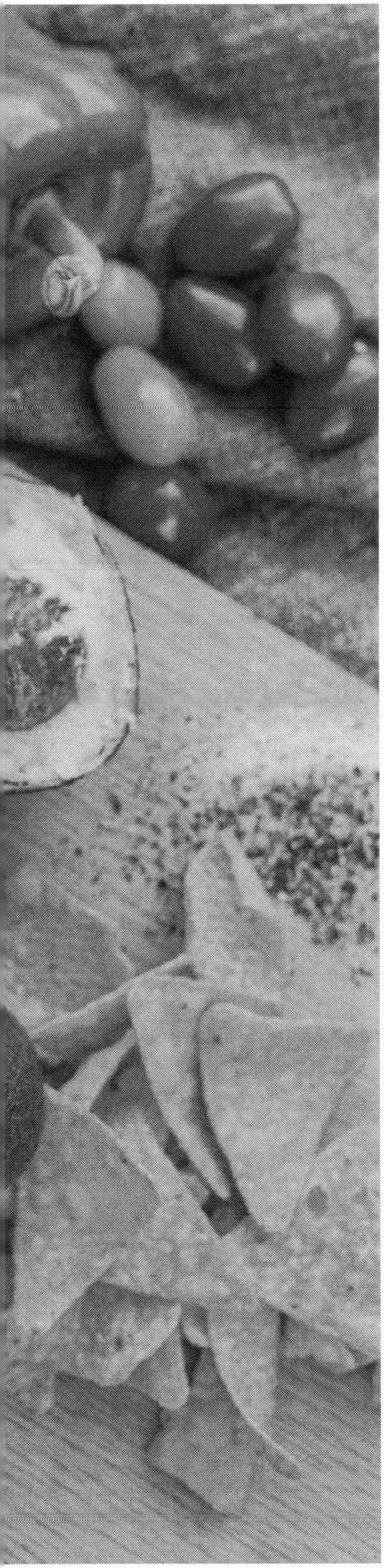

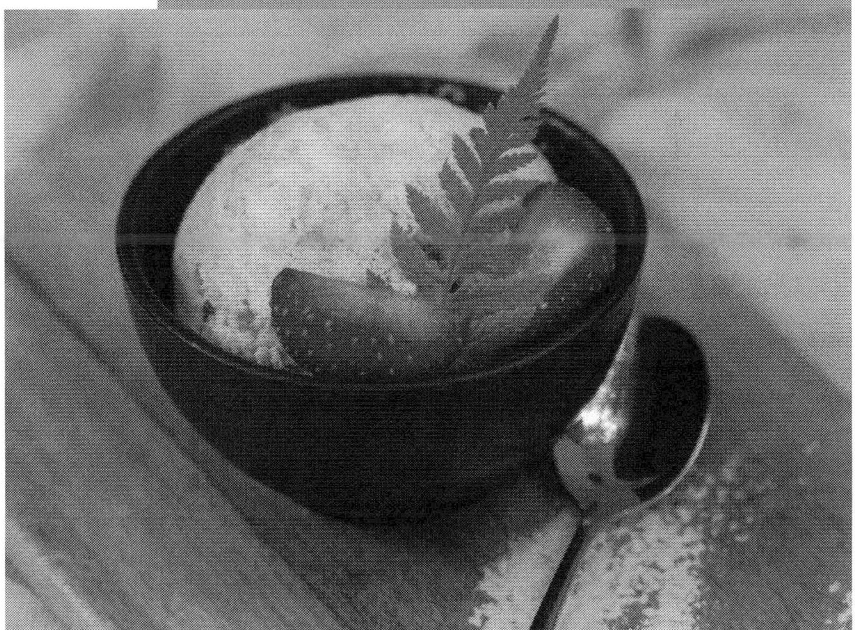

PORTOBELLO MUSHROOMS STUFFED WITH RICOTTA CHEESE

Cooking Difficulty:	Cooking Time:	Servings:
4/10	46 minutes	6

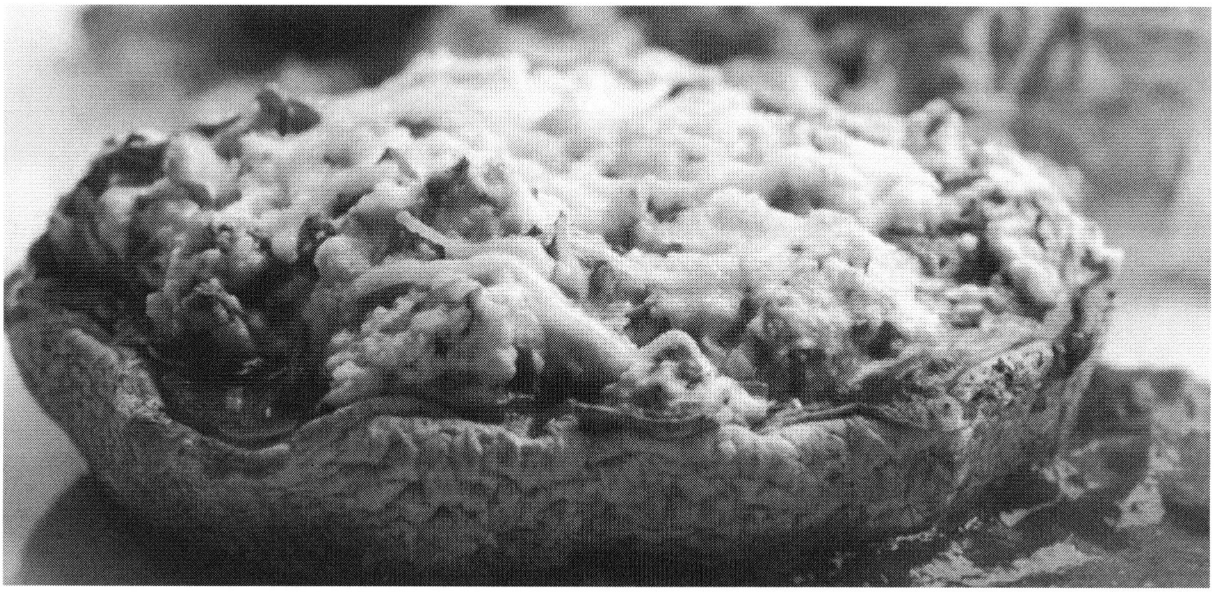

INGREDIENTS

- 6 large portobello mushroom caps
- 3 minced garlic cloves
- 2 small eggs
- 1¼ c. full-fat ricotta cheese
- ¾ c. steamed spinach
- ¾ c. grated parmesan cheese
- ½ c. extra virgin olive oil
- sea salt
- black pepper

NUTRITIONAL INFORMATION

346 Calories, 31.2g Fat, 1.1g Carbs, 15g Protein

STEP 1

Set the oven to 425 degrees F to preheat. Line a baking sheet with aluminum foil and set aside.

STEP 2

Rinse and clean the Portobello mushroom caps thoroughly until all the dirt is washed off. Discard the gills and stems, then blot the mushroom caps with paper towels.

STEP 3

Season the inside of the mushroom caps with salt and pepper, then arrange on the prepared baking sheet.

STEP 4

Bake the mushroom caps for 15 minutes.

STEP 5

Meanwhile, combine the rest of the ingredients in a large bowl until completely combined. Set aside.

STEP 6

Remove the mushroom caps out of the oven and then divide the filling among them. Return to the oven and bake for an additional 25 minutes, or until the mushrooms are browned and tender.

STEP 7

Place the stuffed mushroom caps on a cooling rack and allow to cool slightly. Serve warm.

STEP 8

Store in an airtight container and refrigerate for up to 3 days. Reheat in the microwave oven before serving.

BACON-JALAPENO POPPERS

Cooking Difficulty: 3/10	Cooking Time: 20 minutes	Servings: 12

INGREDIENTS

- 25 jalapeno peppers, fresh
- 2 c. shredded cheddar cheese
- 16 oz. cream cheese
- 32 oz. chopped bacon

STEP 1

Cut the stems of the jalapeño peppers and then cut them lengthwise; remove the seeds.

STEP 2

Fill each with the cream cheese, sprinkle the top with the cheddar cheese, and wrap each cheese-stuffed jalapeño with bacon.

STEP 3

Place on baking sheets, and bake for about 10-15 minutes in a 450F preheated oven, or until the bacon is cooked thoroughly.

STEP 4

Kill the heat and allow to cool; and serve.

NUTRITIONAL INFORMATION

68 Calories, 5.4g Fat, 2.3g Carbs, 2.9g Protein

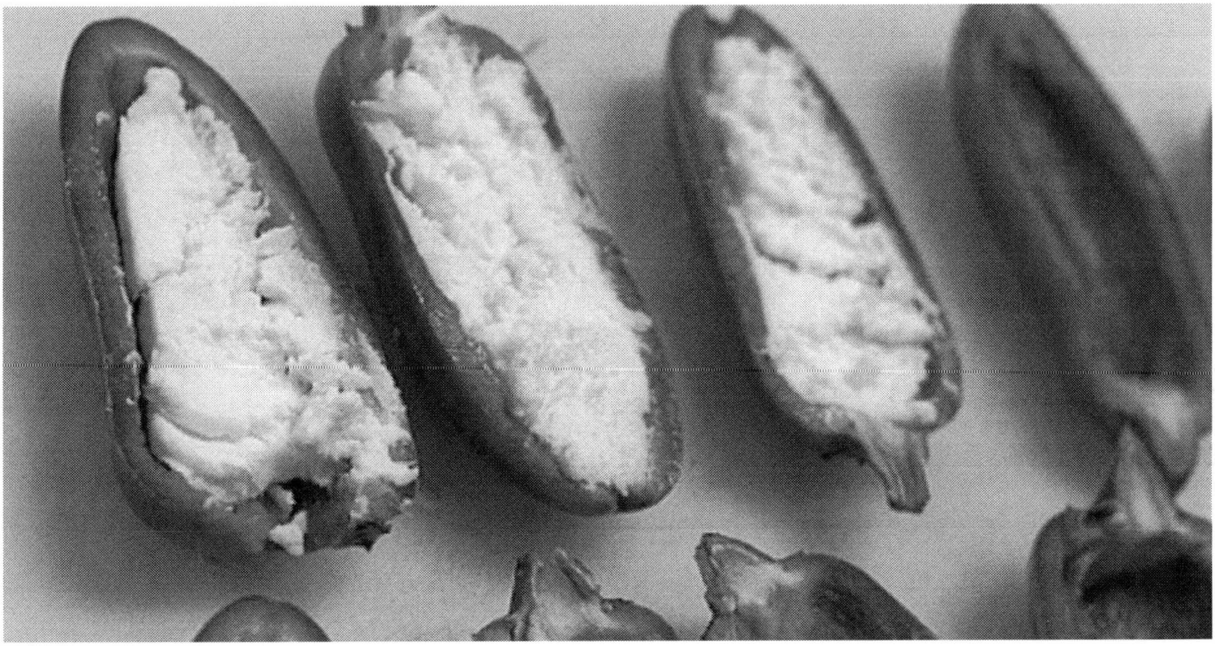

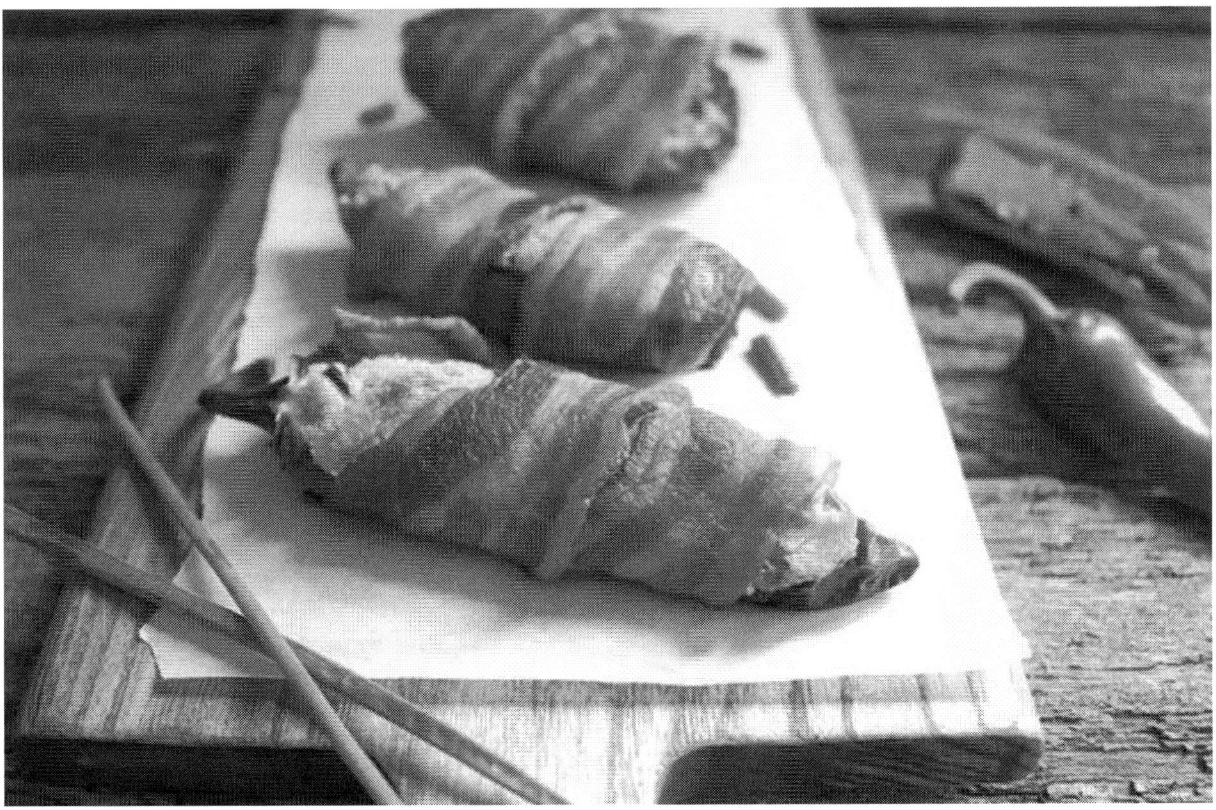

APPLE DETOX

Cooking Difficulty: 1/10	Cooking Time: 2 minutes	Servings: 3

INGREDIENTS

- 1 tsp. honey
- 1tbsp. flax seeds
- ½ apple
- 1½ chopped celery
- 1½ chopped kale
- 1/3 c. ice
- 1/8 c. almond milk

STEP 1

Chop up the apple, celery, and kale. Add these into a blender along with the rest of the ingredients.

STEP 2

Blend until these are mixed well, pour into glasses, and serve.

NUTRITIONAL INFORMATION

50 Calories, 12 g Fats, 5.7g Net Carbs, 16g Protein

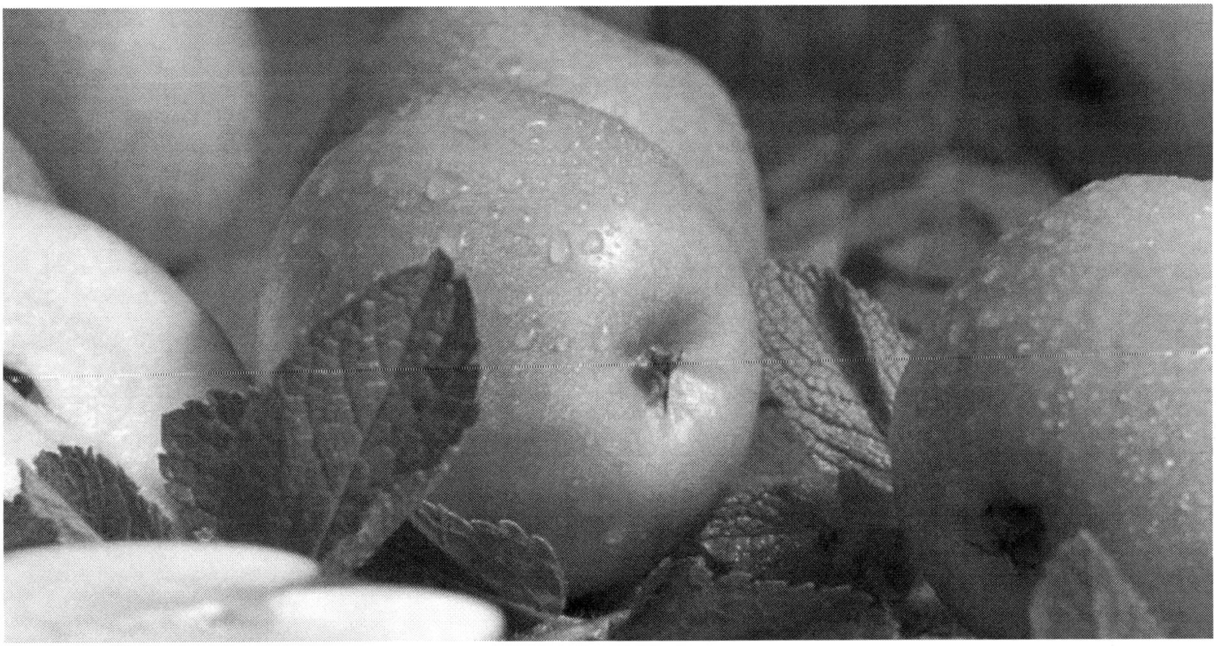

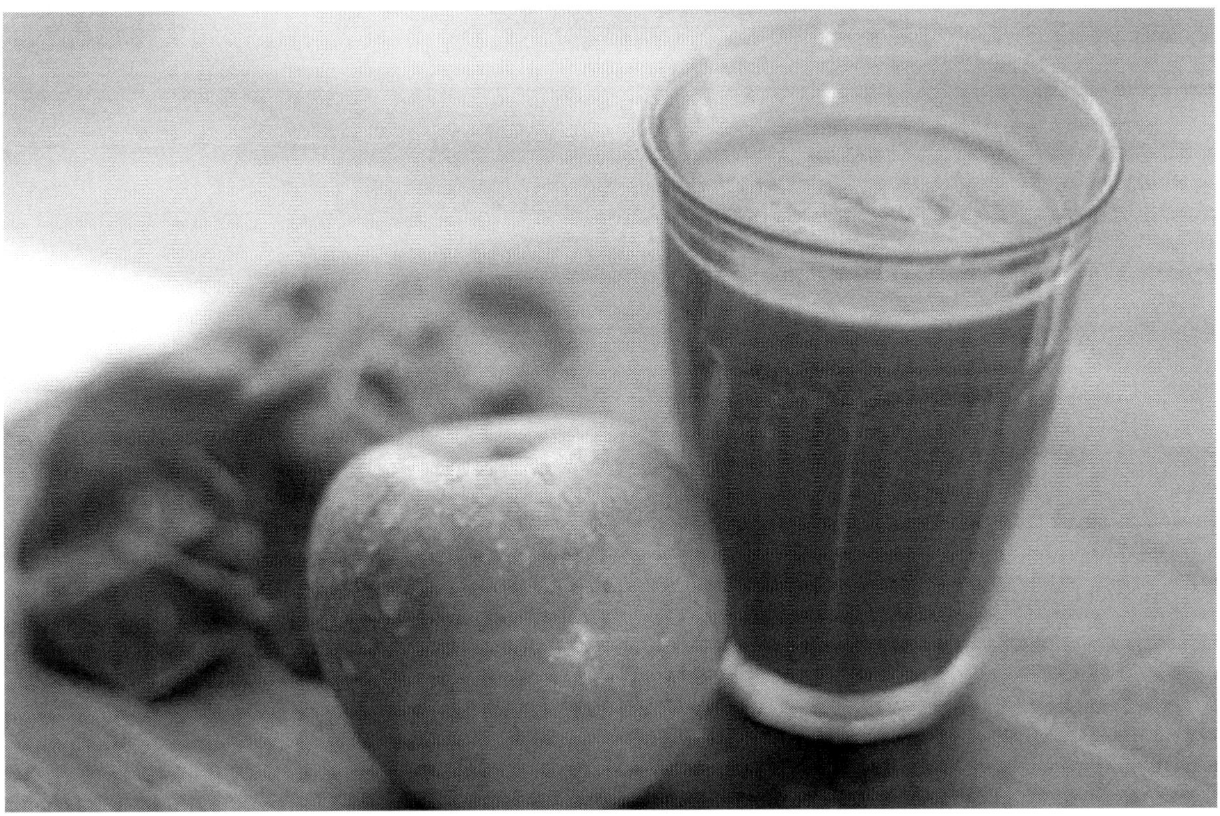

COCONUT MILK ICE CREAM

Cooking Difficulty: 1/10	Cooking Time: 2 minutes	Servings: 5

INGREDIENTS

- 2 cans of coconut milk
- 7 tbsps. cocoa powder
- 7 tbsps. powdered sweetener

STEP 1

Drain the water from the coconut milk cans and reserve only the fats from the top.

STEP 2

Mix in the cocoa and the sweetener.

STEP 3

Put in a container and place it in the quick freeze section of the freezer.

NUTRITIONAL INFORMATION

330 Calories, 30g Fats, 5g Net Carbs, 10g Protein

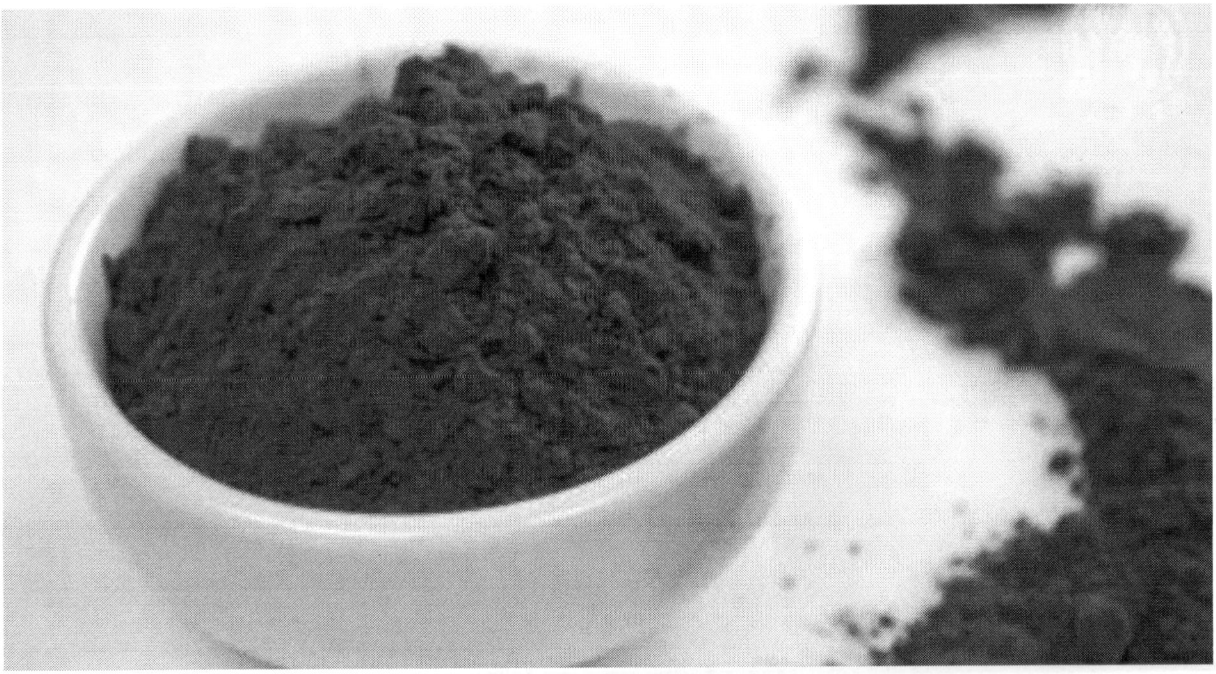

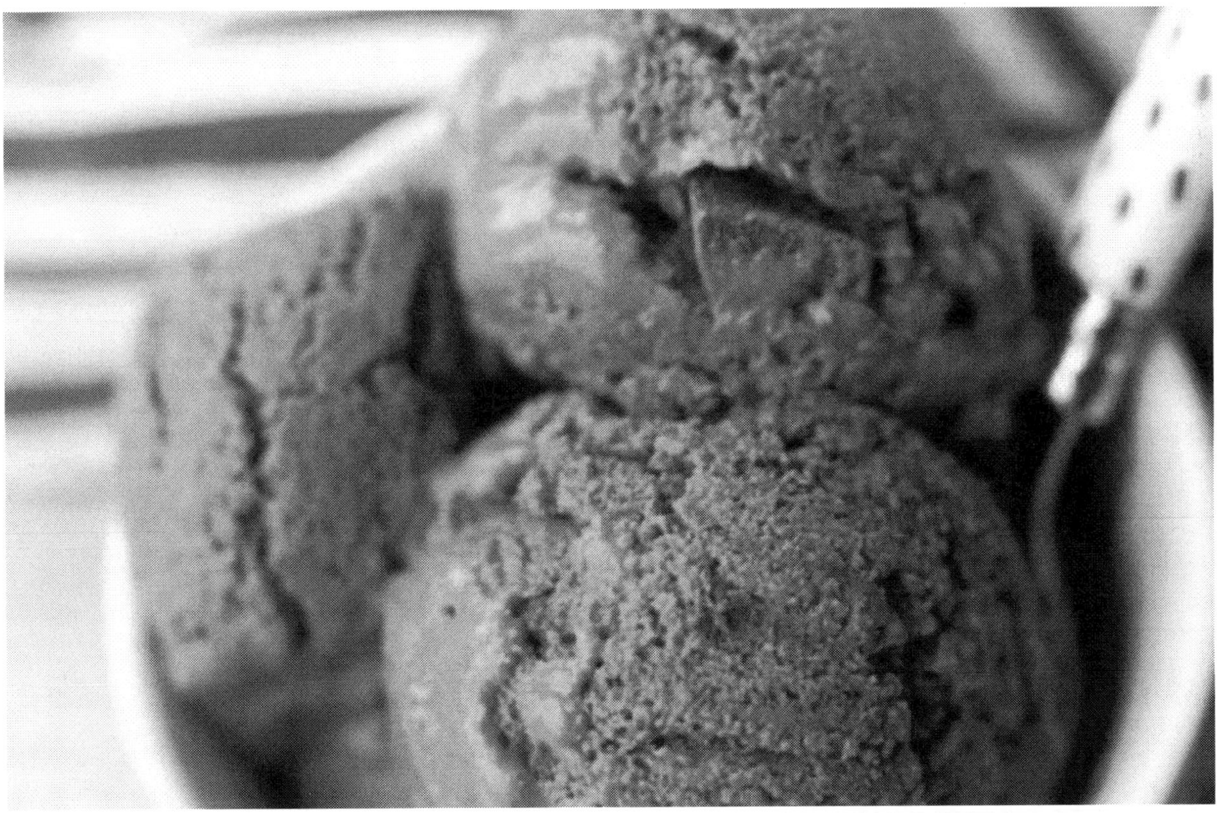

CHEESY CHILI DIP

Cooking Difficulty: 2/10	Cooking Time: 8 minutes	Servings: 8

INGREDIENTS

- 10 oz. kraft old english cheese
- oz. cream cheese
- ½ c. sour cream
- ¼ c. freshly chopped cilantro
- 2 tbsps. minced canned chipotle chili in adobo sauce

STEP 1

In a food processor, blend the English cheese, cream cheese, sour cream, and chipotle until the mixture is soft. Stir in the cilantro, cover, and chill for at least 2 hours before serving.

STEP 2

Serve with assorted sliced vegetables or low carb chips or crackers.

NUTRITIONAL INFORMATION

236 Calories, 12.2g Fat, 3.4g Carbs, 27.1g Protein

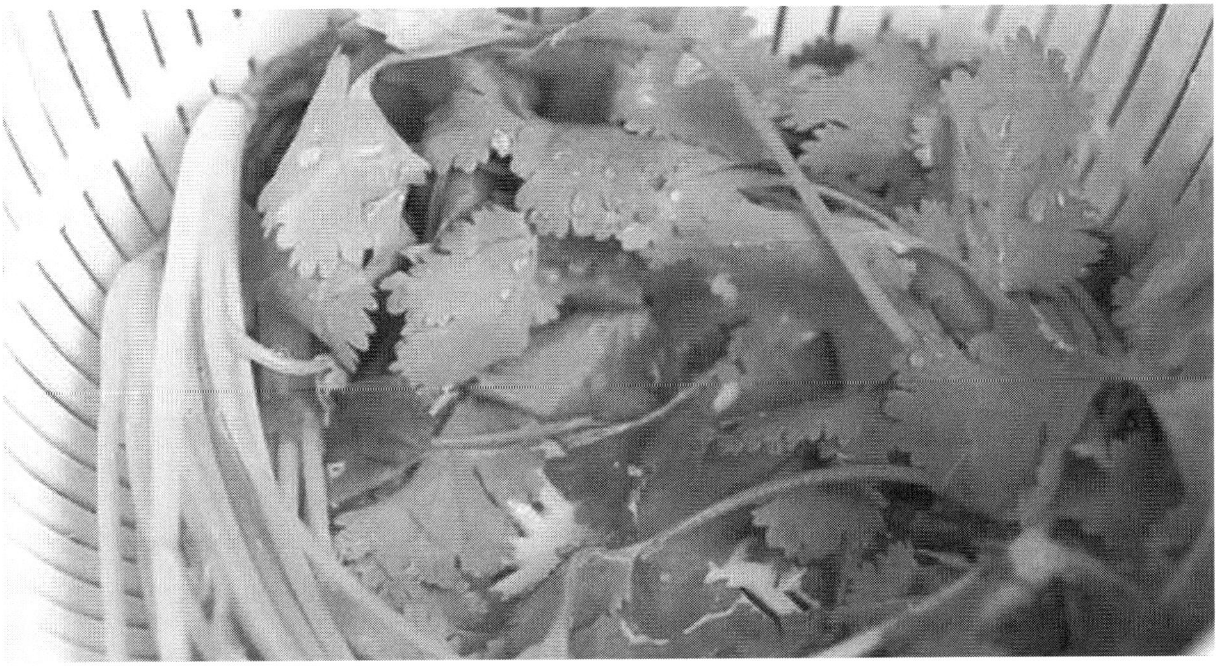

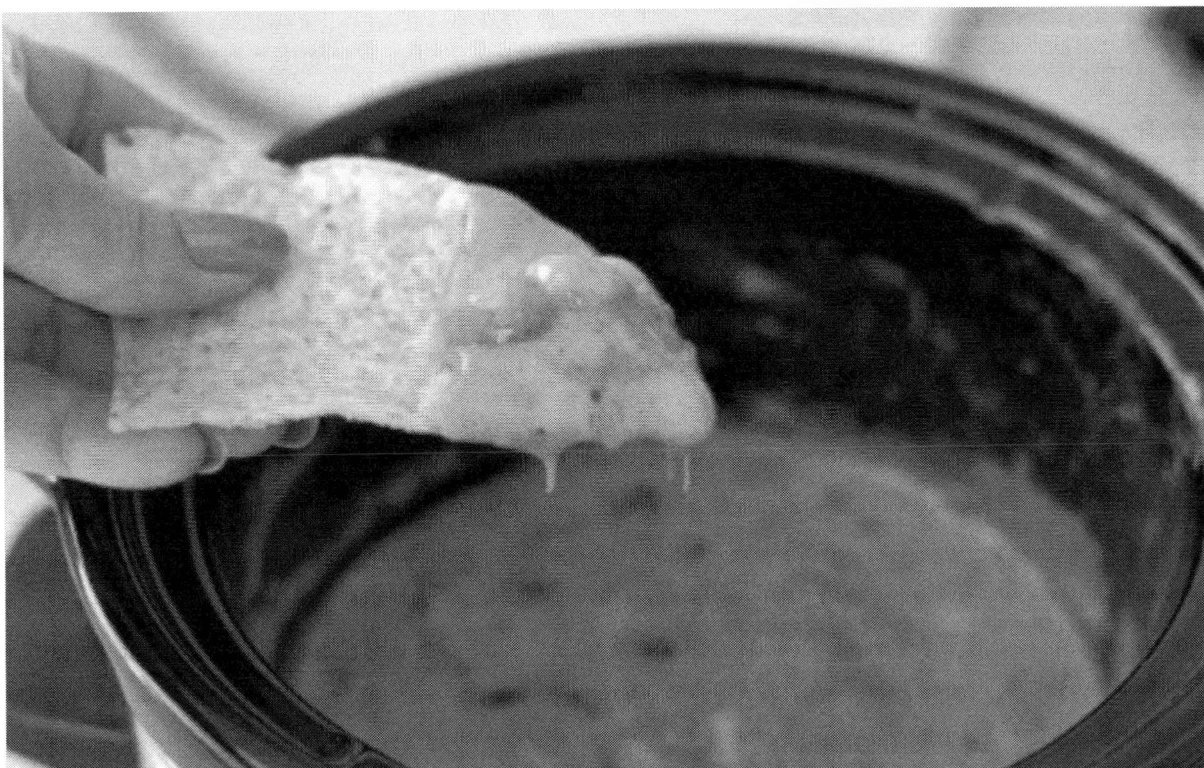

COCONUT CANDY

Cooking Difficulty: 1/10	Cooking Time: 5 minutes	Servings: 18

INGREDIENTS

- 2¼ tsps. stevia
- 1/3 c. coconut milk
- 1½ c. shredded coconut

STEP 1

Combine together the ingredients in a bowl, mixing well.

STEP 2

Pack this down with some plastic wrap and then place it in the fridge for a few hours.

STEP 3

Once it is chilled, scoop the mixture into balls and then place it in a container to store.

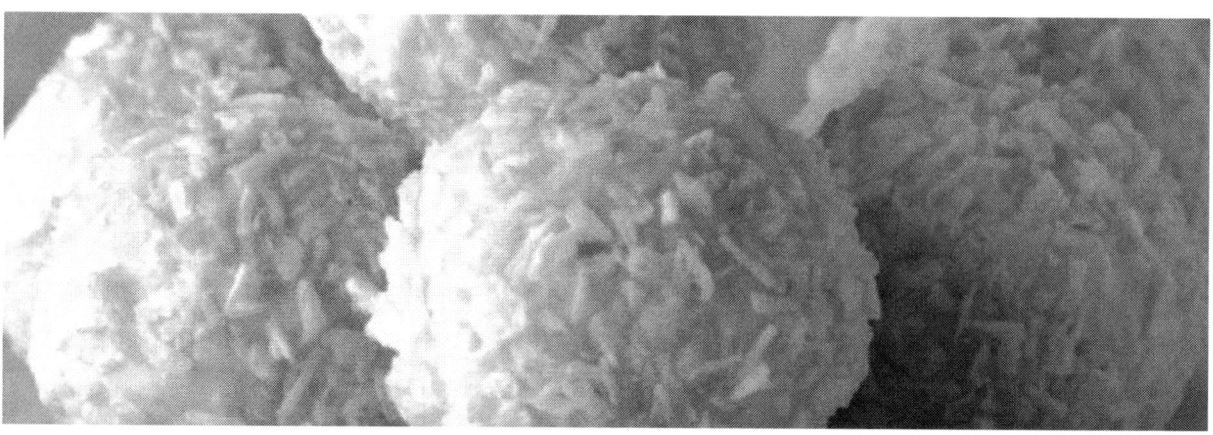

NUTRITIONAL INFORMATION

47 Calories, 5g Fats, 2g Net Carbs, and 4g Protein

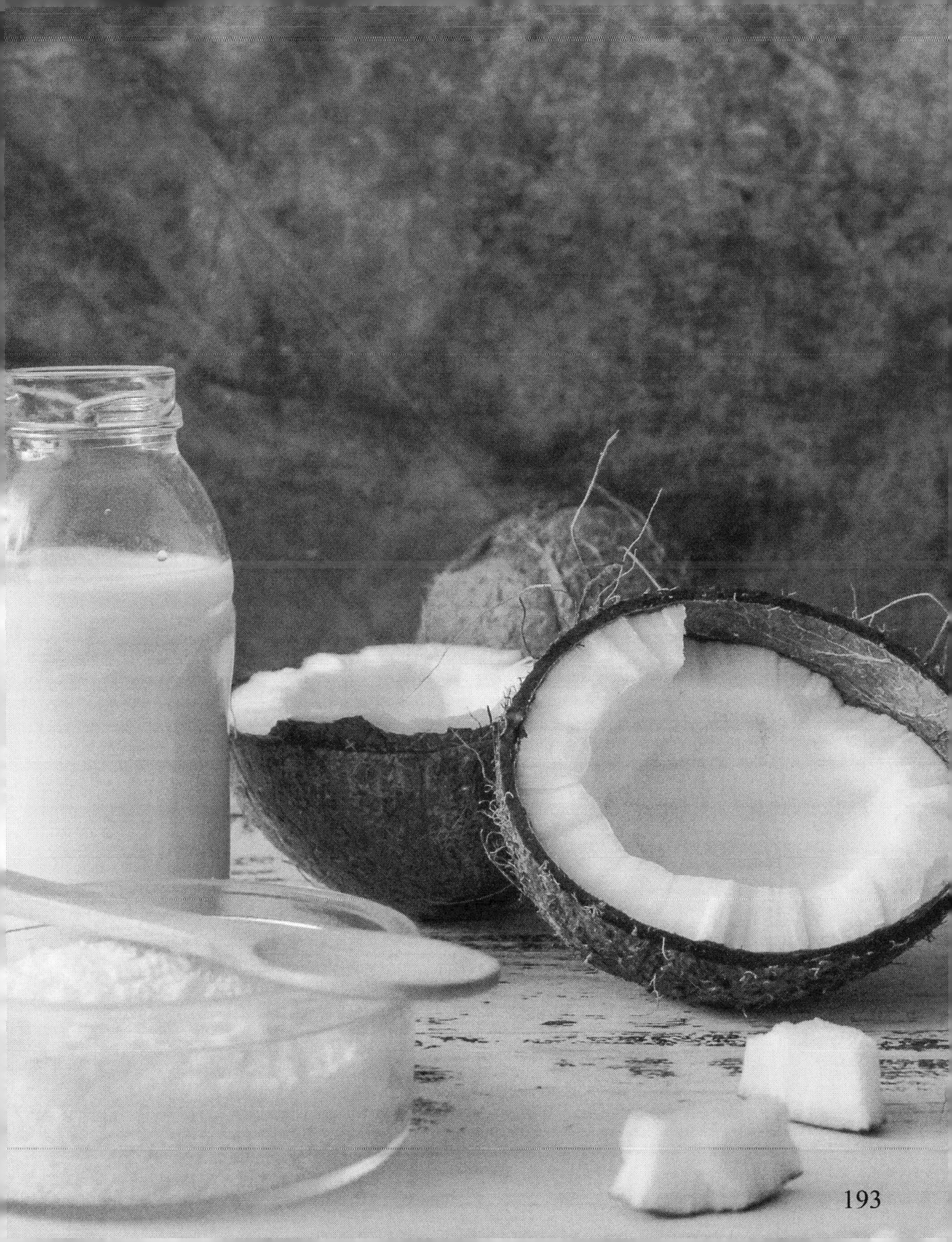

PEANUT BUTTER MOUSSE

Cooking Difficulty: 1/10	Cooking Time: 2 minutes	Servings: 4

INGREDIENTS

- ½ can coconut cream
- tbsps. peanut butter, unsweetened
- 1 tsp. stevia

STEP 1

Combine all ingredients and whip for one minute, until mixture forms peaks.

STEP 2

Chill for at least three hours, or until a mousse texture is achieved.

NUTRITIONAL INFORMATION

206 Calories, 18g Fats, 6g Net Carbs, 5g Protein

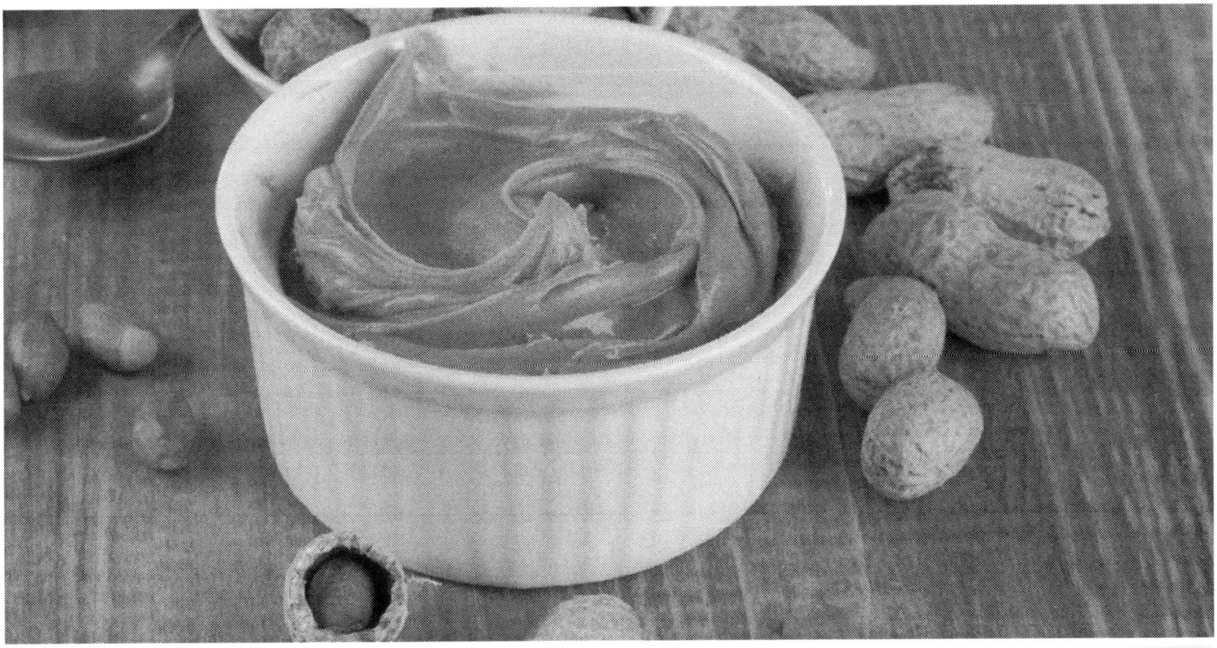

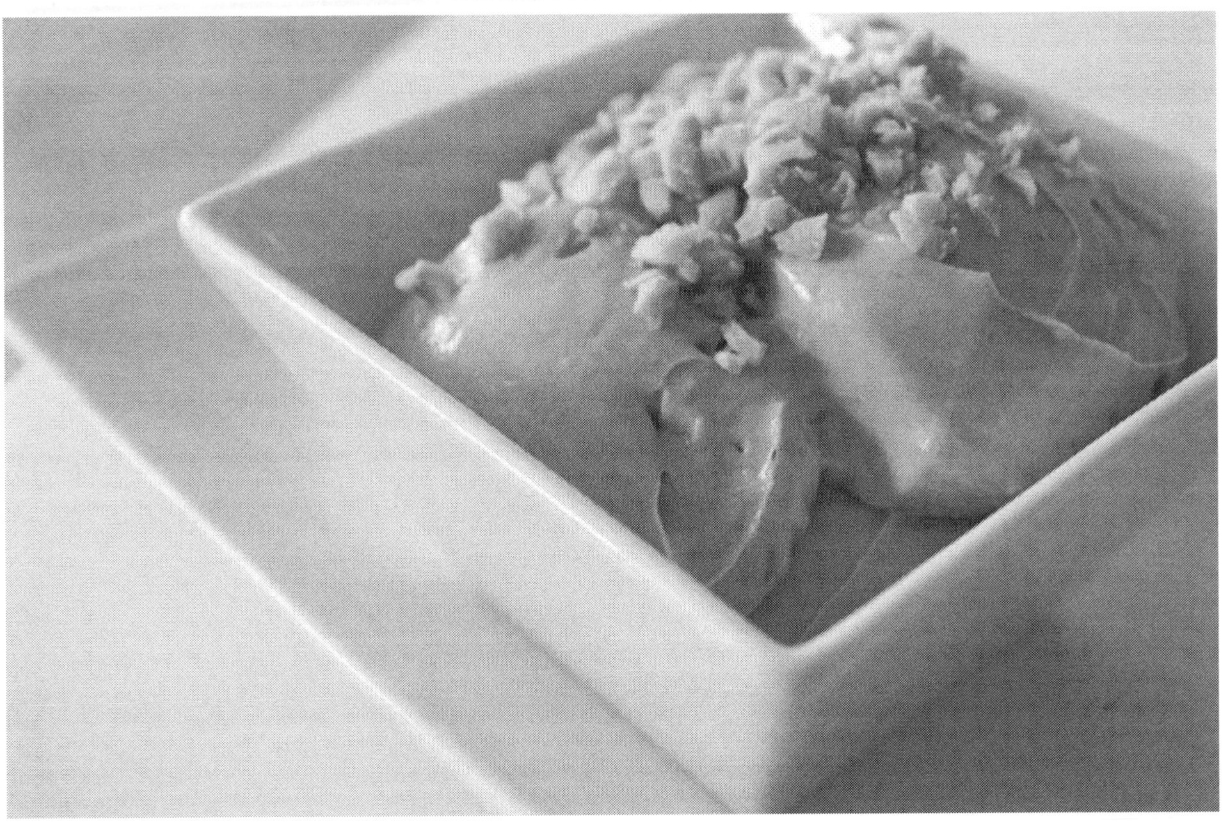

LOW CARB GUACAMOLE

Cooking Difficulty: 1/10	Cooking Time: 4 minutes	Servings: 6

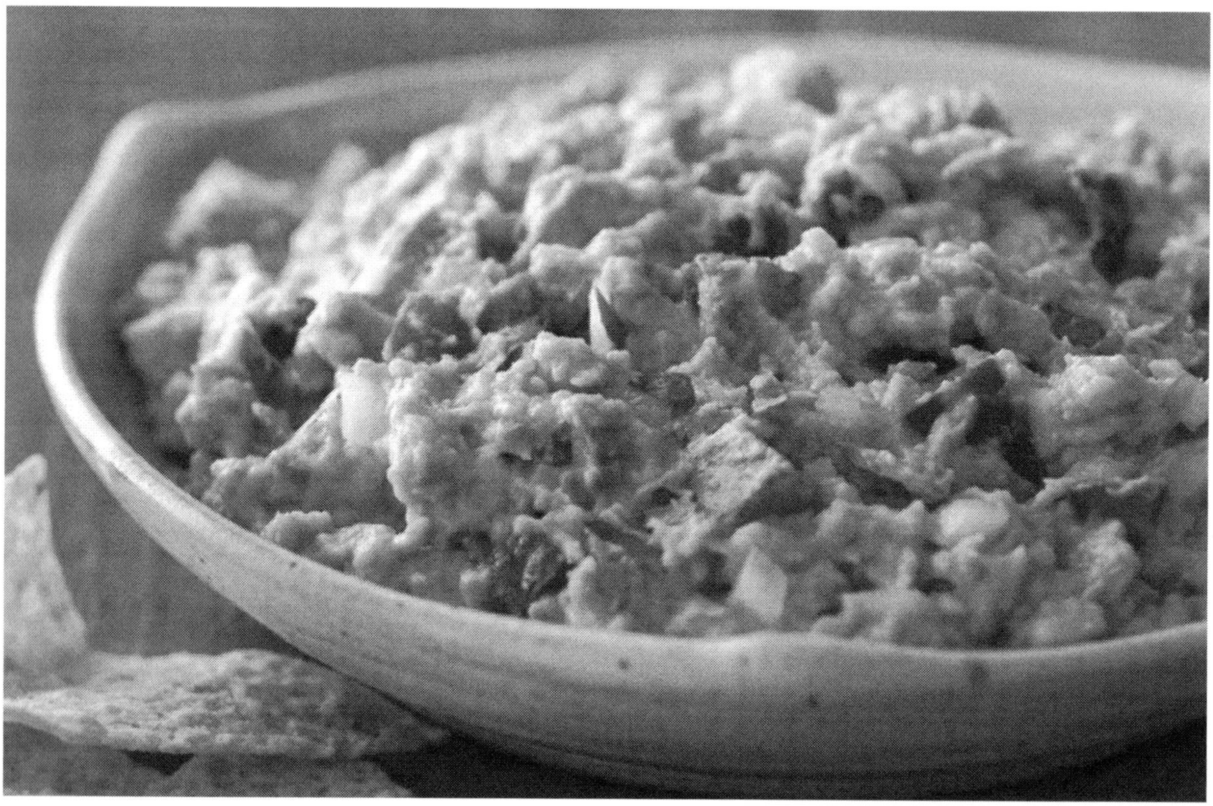

NUTRITIONAL INFORMATION

172 Calories, 15g Fats, 11g Net Carbs, 2g Protein

INGREDIENTS

- 3 large ripe avocados
- 1 diced red onion
- 4 tbsps. squeezed lime juice
- sea salt
- black pepper
- cayenne pepper

STEP 1

Halve the avocados, then discard the stone.

STEP 2

Scoop out the avocado flesh from 3 avocado halves and place them in a large glass bowl. Mash well with a fork or potato masher.

STEP 3

Add 2 tablespoons of lime juice into the mashed avocado and mix well.

STEP 4

Dice the remaining avocado then place it in a separate bowl. Add the remaining lime juice and toss gently to coat.

STEP 5

Combine the diced avocado with the mashed avocado, then add the chopped onion. Toss again to combine.

STEP 6

Season the guacamole with salt, pepper, and cayenne pepper then mix gently to combine.

STEP 7

Store in an airtight container for up to 3 days. Serve with carrot, celery, and cucumber sticks.

SMOKED SALMON AND DILL SPREAD

Cooking Difficulty: 1/10	Cooking Time: 3 minutes	Servings: 6

INGREDIENTS

- 4 oz. smoked salmon
- 4 oz. full fat cream cheese
- 2½ tbsps. mayonnaise
- 2 tbsps. chopped fresh dill
- sea salt
- black pepper

STEP 1

Pour the smoked salmon, mayonnaise, and cream cheese into a food processor. Pulse until combined.

STEP 2

Pour the mixture into an airtight container and mix in the fresh dill. Season to taste with salt and pepper.

STEP 3

Cover and refrigerate for up to 3 days. Best served with carrot, celery, and cucumber sticks.

NUTRITIONAL INFORMATION

50 Calories, 4.8g Fat, 0.31g Carbs, 0.9g Protein

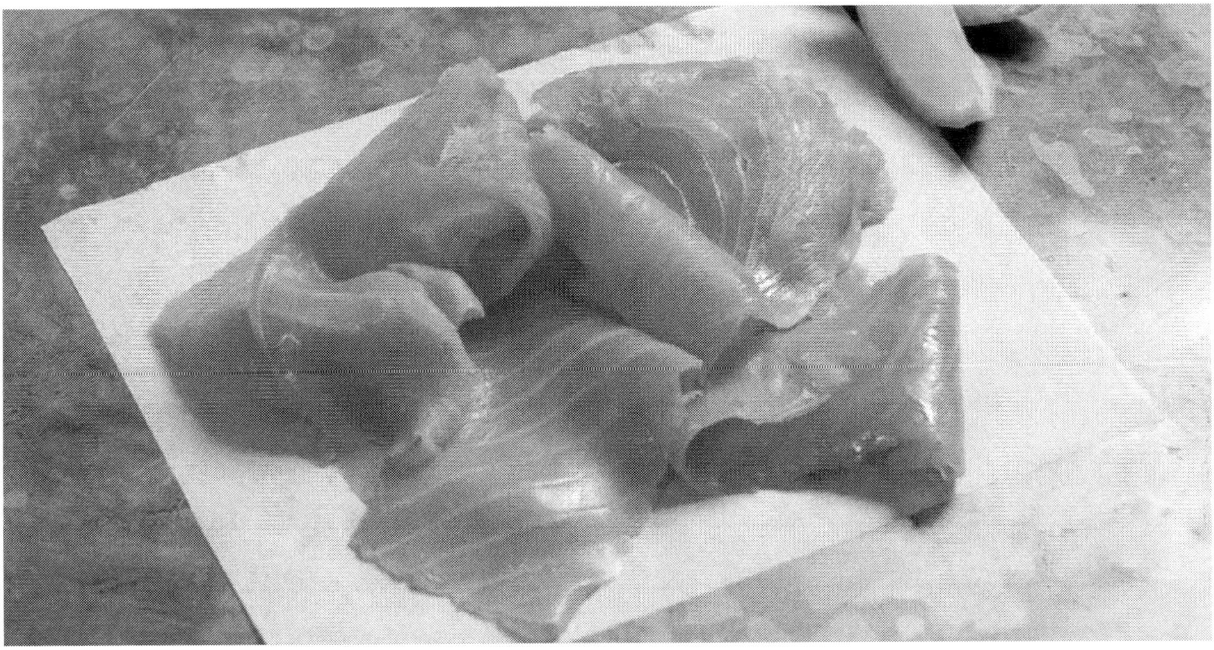

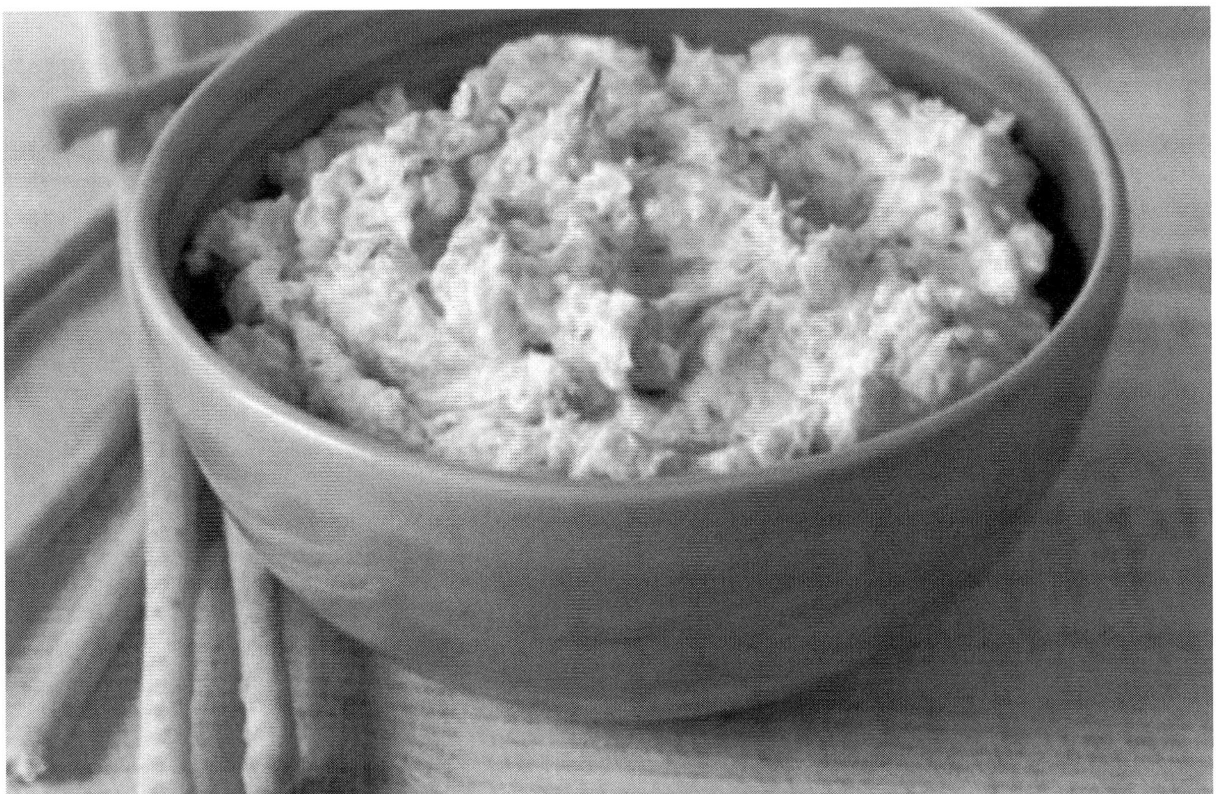

CINNAMON BUTTER

Cooking Difficulty: 2/10	Cooking Time: 12 minutes	Servings: 8

INGREDIENTS

- ½ c. butter
- 5 drops liquid stevia
- ½ tsp. pure vanilla extract
- ½ tsp. ground cinnamon
- 1/8 tsp. fine sea salt

STEP 1

Combine the butter, vanilla, cinnamon, salt, and stevia in a large bowl. Mix well until smooth.

STEP 2

Line a baking sheet with wax paper then spread the cinnamon butter mixture on top. Roll the paper to seal the butter mixture, then seal the ends.

STEP 3

Refrigerate the butter for 1 hour before using. Store in the refrigerator for up to 2 weeks. Best served on the Keto Bread or with celery sticks.

NUTRITIONAL INFORMATION

103 Calories, 12g Fats, 0.1g Net Carbs, 0.1g Protein

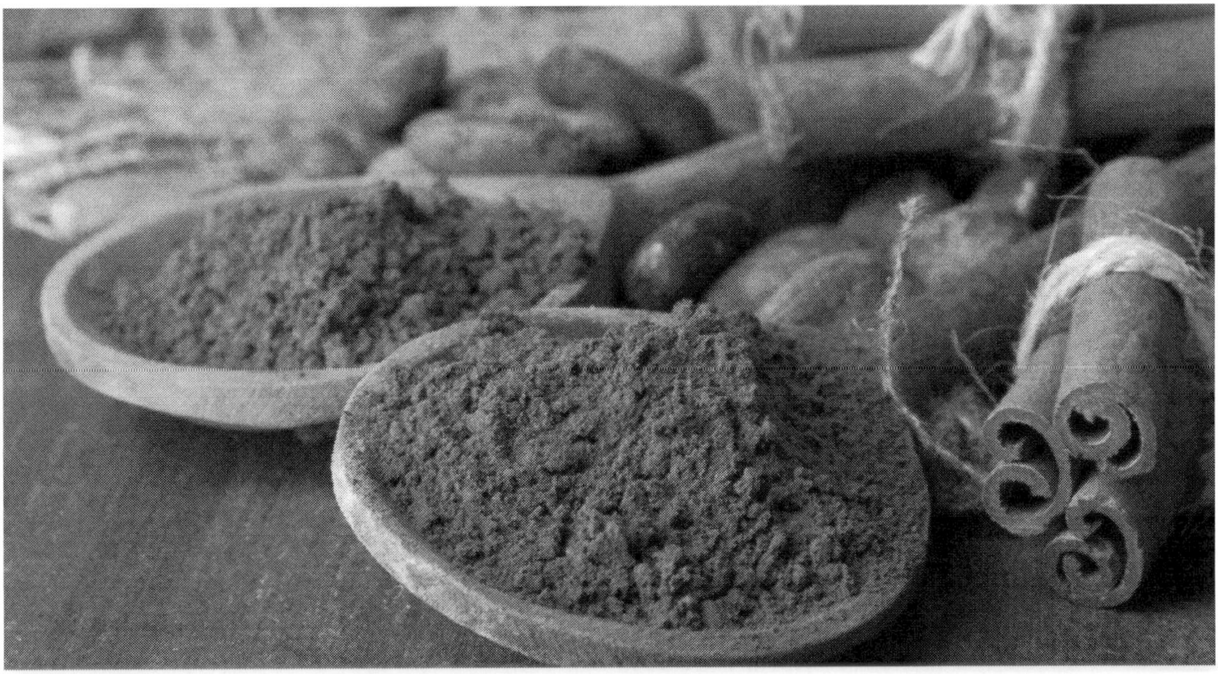

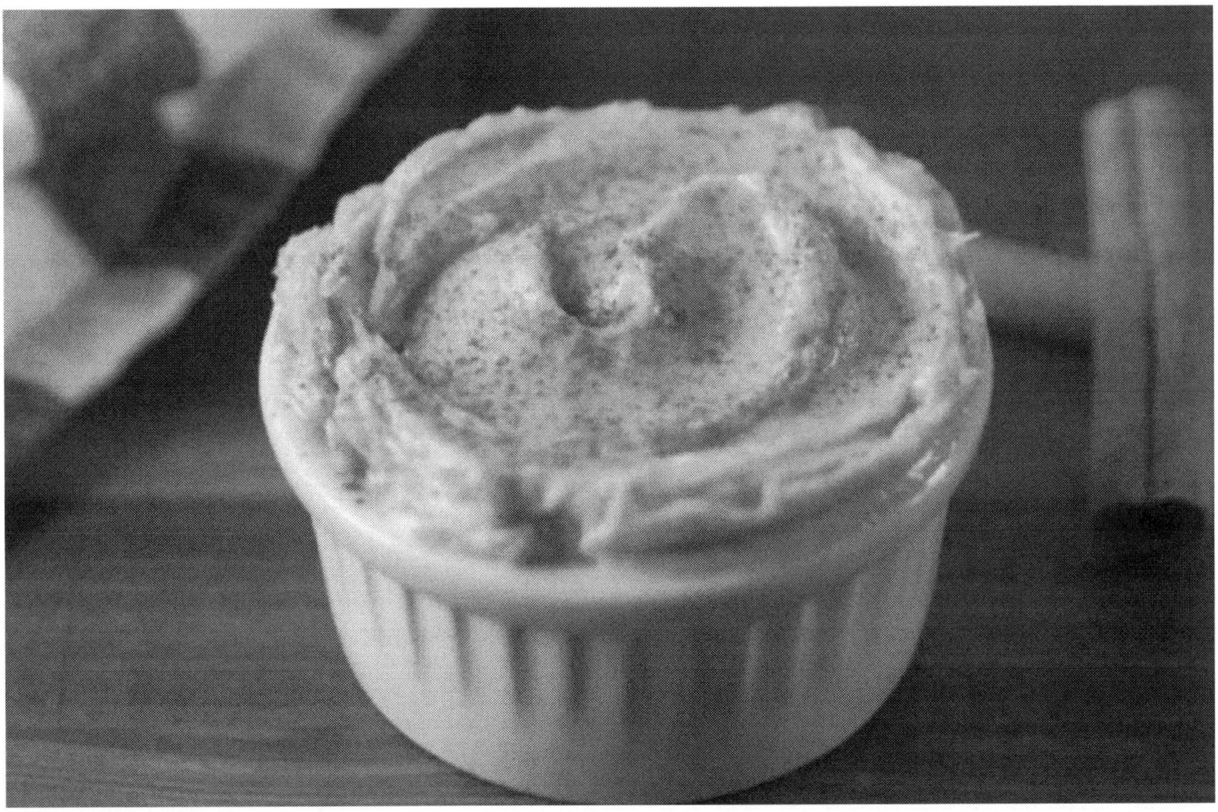

MANGO SMOOTHIE

Cooking Difficulty:	Cooking Time:	Servings:
1/10	2 minutes	1

INGREDIENTS

- 6 ice cubes
- 1 tbsp. sugar
- 1 tbsp. lemon juice
- ¼ c. vanilla yogurt
- ½ c. mango juice
- ¼ c. mashed avocado
- ¼ c. mango cubes

STEP 1

Cut the mango into cubes. Cube up the avocado as well.

STEP 2

Take out the blender and add all of the ingredients together. Blend until smooth and then serve.

NUTRITIONAL INFORMATION

269 Calories, 9 g Fats, 6 g Net Carbs, and 4g Protein

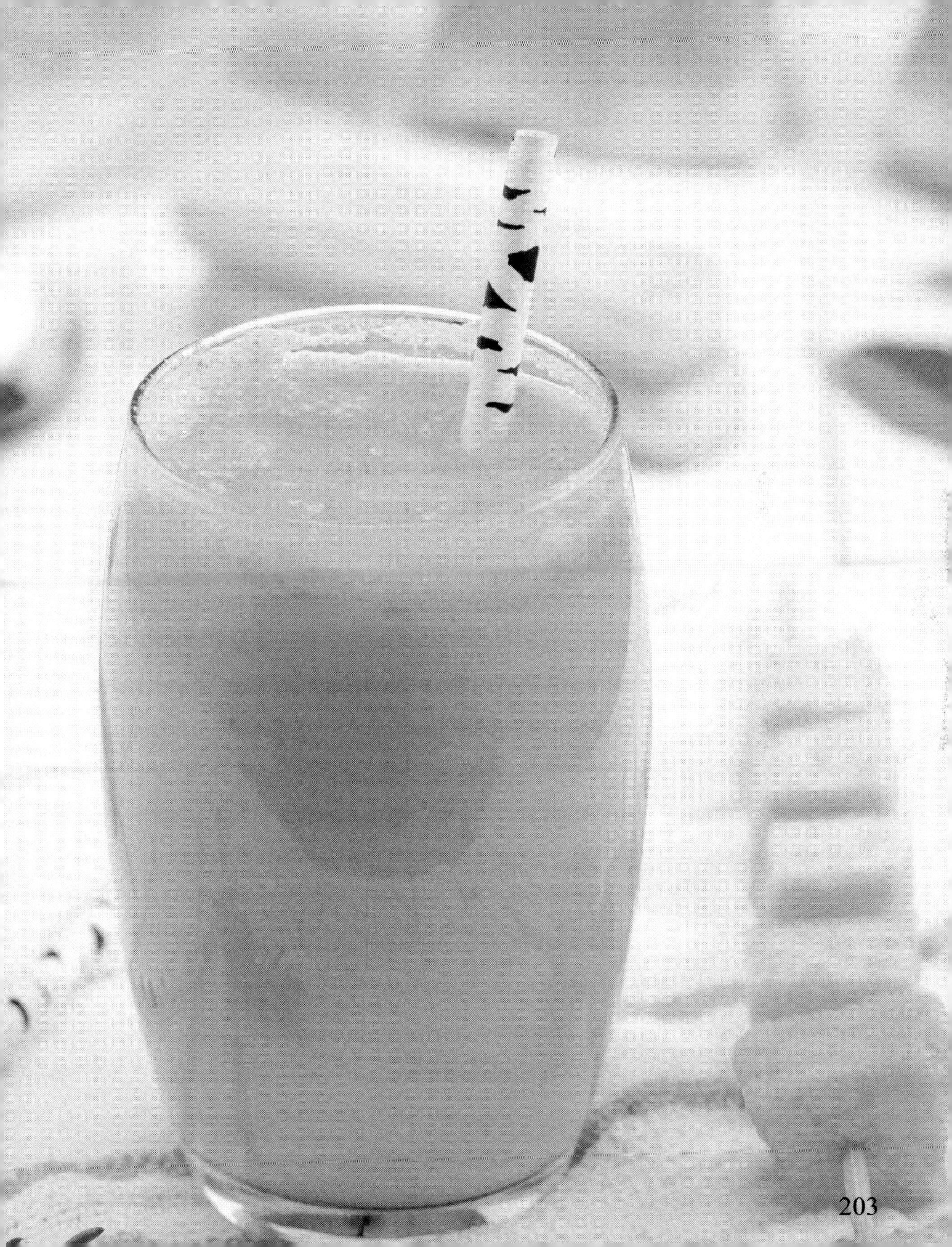

RASPBERRY POPS

Cooking Difficulty: 2/10	Cooking Time: 6 minutes	Servings: 8

INGREDIENTS

- 1 tsp. vanilla
- 4 tbsps. butter
- 4 tbsps. heavy cream
- 4 tbsps. coconut oil
- ¼ c. chopped raspberries
- ¼ c. cream cheese

STEP 1

Combine butter, coconut oil and cream cheese. Preheat them in the microwave.

STEP 2

Remove bowl from microwave and stir. Add heavy cream and fold the raspberries.

STEP 3

Stir the vanilla and make sure everything is well mixed. Pour into an ice cream pan and place in the freezer.

STEP 4

Let them cool down until they freeze.

NUTRITIONAL INFORMATION

166 Calories, 17 g Fats, 2g Net Carbs, and 8g Protein

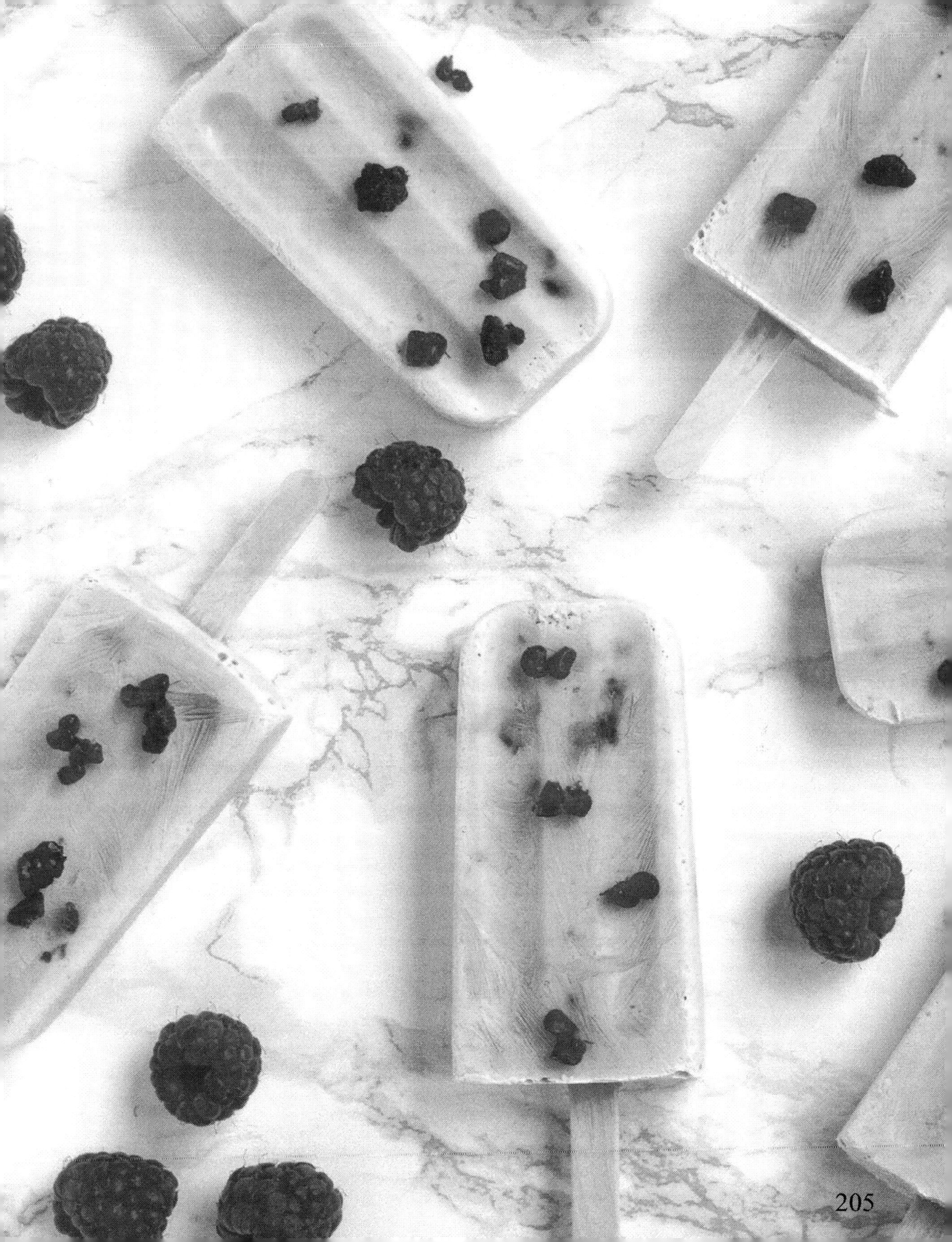

KETO LAVA CAKE

Cooking Difficulty: 2/10	Cooking Time: 16 minutes	Servings: 1

INGREDIENTS

- ½ tsp. vanilla
- 1 tbsp. heavy cream
- 1 egg
- 2 tbsps. erythritol
- 2 tbsps. cocoa powder
- salt
- ¼ tsp. baking powder

STEP 1

Allow the oven to heat up to 350 degrees. While that heats up, bring out a bowl and whisk together the erythritol and cocoa powder.

STEP 2

In a second bowl, beat the egg. Add this into the erythritol mixture along with the rest of the ingredients.

STEP 3

Prepare a few ramekins before adding in the batter. Place into the oven to bake.

STEP 4

After 15 minutes, take the cakes out and let them cool down before enjoying them.

NUTRITIONAL INFORMATION

173 Calories, 13 g Fats, 4g Net Carbs, and 8g Protein

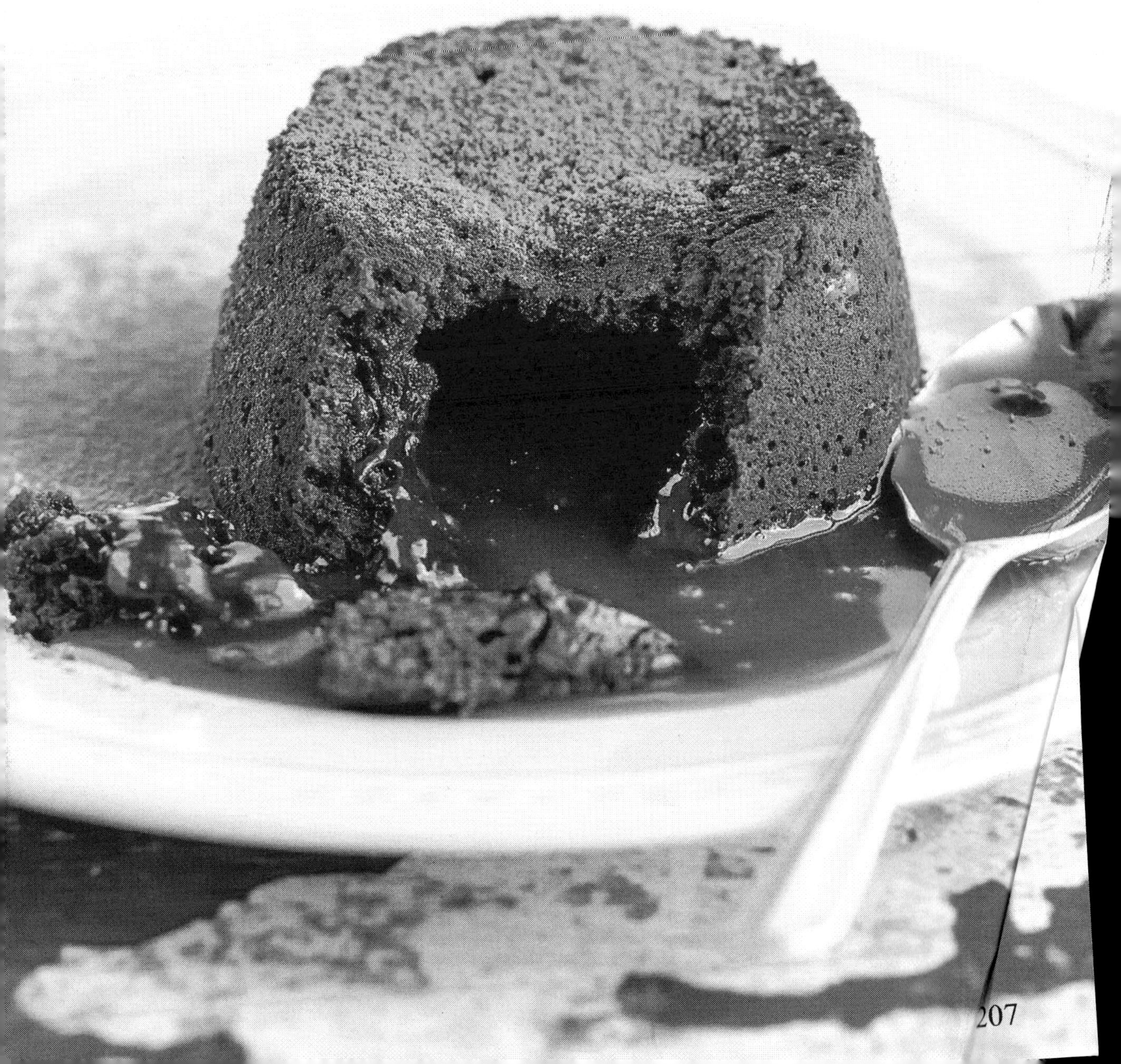

BLACKBERRY CHEESECAKE SMOOTHIE

Cooking Difficulty:	Cooking Time:	Servings:
1/10	2 minutes	1

INGREDIENTS

- 6 ice cubes
- sweetener
- ¾ c. coconut milk
- ¼ tsp. vanilla extract
- 1 tsp. coconut oil
- ¼ c. frozen blackberries
- ¼ c. water

STEP 1

Cream the coconut milk: This is a simple process. All you need to do is place the can of coconut milk in the refrigerator overnight. The next morning, open the can and spoon out the coconut milk that has solidified. Don't shake the can before opening. Discard the liquids.

STEP 2

Add all of the ingredients, save the ice cubes, to the blender, and blend on low speed until pureed. Thin with water as needed.

STEP 3

Add in the ice cubes and blend until the smoothie reaches your desired consistency.

NUTRITIONAL INFORMATION

328 Calories, 7g Net Carbs, 12g Fats, 8g Protein

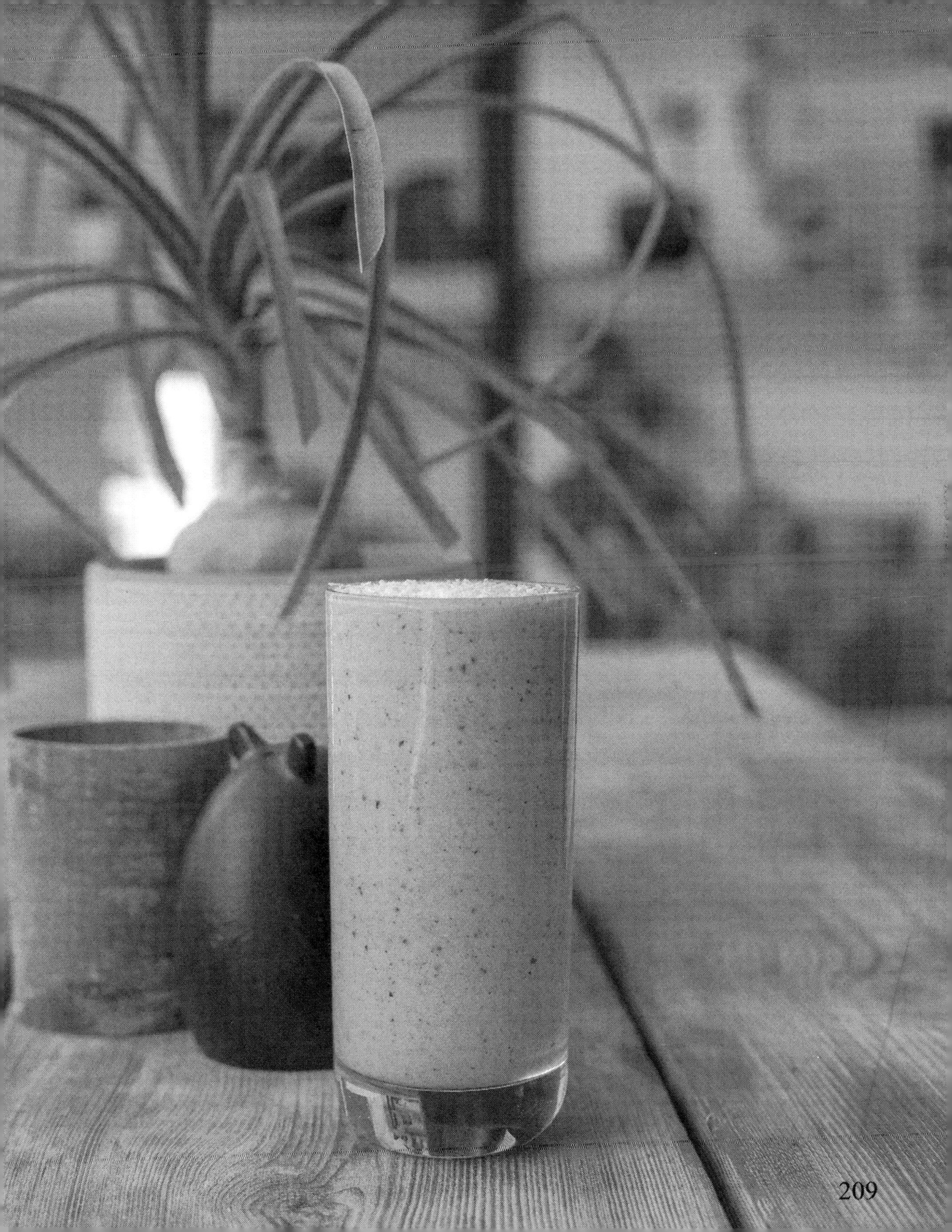

CONCLUSION

I do hope that this book has been helpful and you found the information contained within the chapters useful!

For those who have already been able to make the mental conversion to change, then I trust that you will find this a far more accessible and easy to maintain eating method than those you may have tackled in the past. I am convinced that just a few weeks on the Ketogenic diet will produce such good results that you will be encouraged to turn it into a permanent way of life.

Keep in mind that you are not only limited to the recipes provided in this book! Just go ahead and keep on exploring until you create your very own culinary masterpiece!

Stay healthy and stay safe!

Jerry Carr

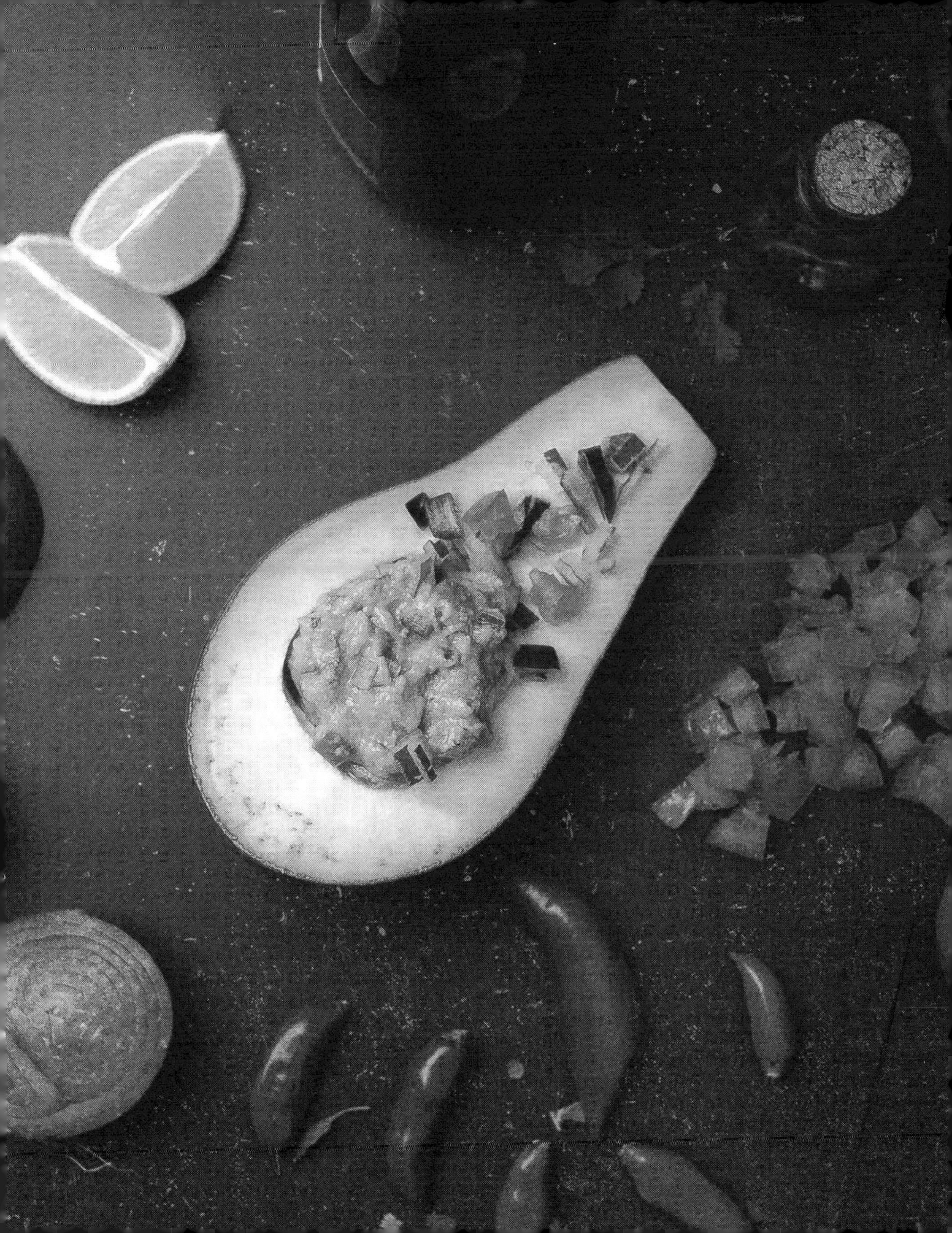

Printed in Great Britain
by Amazon

62493927R00120